Self-management of Long-term Health Conditions

A Handbook for People with Chronic Disease

NHS Expert Patients Programme

BULL PUBLISHING COMPANY
BOULDER, COLORADO USA

Copyright © 2002 Bull Publishing Company

ISBN 0-923521-74-7

Bull Publishing Company
P.O. Box 1377
Boulder, Colorado 80306
(303) 545-6350
(303) 545-6354 (fax)
www.bullpub.com

Supported by AHCPR Grant HSO 6680 and California State Tobacco-Related Disease Research Program Award 1RT 156

Library of Congress Cataloging-in-Publication Data (US edition)

Living a healthy life with chronic conditions: self-management of arthritis, asthma, bronchitis, diabetes, emphysema, heart disease. multiple sclerosis, and others / Kate Lorig . . . [et al.].— English Edition.
    p.cm.
    Includes bibliographical references and index.
    ISBN 0-923521-74-7
    1. Chronic diseases—Popular works. 2. Medicine, Popular. I. Lorig, Kate

    RC108.L565 2000
    616'.044—dc21   00-022528

Publisher: James Bull
Cover Design: Department of Health, England
Interior Design and Composition: Shadow Canyon Graphics
Illustrations: Publication Services
Editing and Proofreading: see section on Acknowledgments

SELF-MANAGEMENT OF LONG-TERM HEALTH CONDITIONS
A Handbook for People with Chronic Disease

This handbook draws on the material in the US Second Edition of "Living a Healthy Life with Chronic Conditions" by Kate Lorig, Halsted Holman, David Sobel, Diana Laurent, Virginia Gonzalez, Marian Minor and Peg Harrison.

Keeping to the integrity of the US edition, Chapters 1-3 and 9 have been revised for UK users of the handbook. Some of the other chapters have been suitably modified. Disease-specific supplements commissioned by the Department of Health, England, will be issued separately to the handbook. These replace Chapters 9, 15, 16, 17 and 18 in the US edition. The handbook will be an evolving document. As users in the UK provide feedback on the handbook, changes may be made to it as necessary.

TABLE OF CONTENTS

v

ACKNOWLEDGMENTS TO THE UK EDITION

We deeply appreciate the readiness of the authors and publisher of the original US edition, in particular Kate Lorig and Jim Bull, to support the NHS Expert Patients Programme in England and also wish to thank them for encouraging the preparation of this handbook designed specifically for use in England. A number of people in the UK have helped in its preparation. Jean Thompson and Jim Phillips contributed extensively to the original as well as the UK editions. Douglas Brown worked to ensure the spellings and phrases were in UK English. A number of advisors at the Department of Health in England helped revise the text. Roy Jones co-ordinated and contributed to these revisions. Jim Phillips revised Chapter 9. Anne Kennedy, Dr Vivienne Press and Ayesha Dost provided guidance on all the chapters. Anne Kennedy also revised the first three chapters. Jean Thompson and Jim Phillips contributed to the background on the Expert Patients Programme. We wish to thank all these individuals for their valuable contributions.

A number of others contributed to the development of the disease-specific supplements. Their contribution and support will be acknowledged separately in the supplements as and when they are published.

vi

ACKNOWLEDGMENTS TO THE ORIGINAL US EDITION

Many people have helped us write this book. Among the most important are the first 1000 participants of the Stanford University Chronic Disease Self-Management study. These have been followed by thousands of other course participants in the United States, Australia, New Zealand, Canada, and Great Britain. All of these people, along with our wonderful course leaders, have told us what information they needed and helped us make adjustments as we went along.

There are also many professionals who have assisted us: Susan Kayman, Suephy Chen, Sandra Wilson, Margo Harris, Nancy Brannigan, Jim Phillips, Jean Thompson, Lynne Newcombe, John Lynch, Mary Hobbs, Marty Klein, Nazanin Dashtara, Vivian Vestal, María Hernández-Marin, Richard Rubio, and Laurie Doyle. To all of you, your help has been greatly received. A special thanks to Gloria Samuel, who kept us all on track and put this book together.

Finally, thanks to David Bull to whom this book is dedicated. David was our first publisher and had faith in this project that allowed us to proceed. Without him, there may never have been a book. His son Jim has continued the family tradition with support and encouragement for this second edition.

To David Bull,
who made this book possible

INTRODUCTION BY THE CHIEF MEDICAL OFFICER

The Expert Patients Programme is about creating a partnership between doctor and patient, and giving patients the skills to become equal partners and take over some of the management of their own illness. We plan, over time, to make this an integral part of NHS provision for the 17 million people living with chronic conditions in Great Britain. Expert Patients have been shown to make more effective, focused use of health and social services. The bottom line is that they feel their quality of life is improved—they have control rather than being dominated by their disease.

The Expert Patients Programme will help to create a new generation of patients who are empowered to take action in partnership with the health professional caring for them, for example, to reduce pain, to improve the use of medication, and enhance their overall quality of life. Patients will receive the support to help them take more control of their own health and treatment, to make more appropriate use of health and social services, and become more empowered.

Liam Donaldson
Chief Medical Officer for England

ORIGINS OF THIS HANDBOOK AND THE EXPERT PATIENTS PROGRAMME

Occupational therapists, doctors, nurses and other heath and social care professionals have for many years attempted to help patients develop abilities in managing their own health. In some parts of the world these efforts have led to the development of methods of training people in self-management of their health. Some of these approaches may be led through partnerships between professionals and knowledgeable patients, and others are led by lay individuals who have become experts in the management of their own conditions through years of experience of living with one as well as by having gone through structured training to manage their own condition.

A lay-led structured training programme was pioneered by Professor Kate Lorig of Stanford University, USA. In the 1970s Kate Lorig produced an initial practical approach to self-management and then in the 1980s based it on Stanford Professor of Social Psychology Albert Bandura's work on social learning. Their first courses were based on the experiences of people with arthritis.

Arthritis Care used this method in the UK for patients with arthritis. A handful of other agencies in the UK helped provide self-management training courses for a variety of other chronic disease groups. The Long-term Medical Conditions Alliance coordinated a project for nine voluntary organisations to deliver the course. In the UK, as elsewhere, lay-led self-management courses have proved to be an effective way of training people with long-term conditions to take an active role in the management of their lives.

A literature search commissioned by the Department of Health and done by Coventry University suggested that there were a huge number of studies looking into the effects of self-management training. The studies indicate that there is substantial international research evidence to show that training in self-management of long-term illness leads to a large number of beneficial effects in terms of improvement in the quality of life of the patient as well as reduction in use of health and social care services.

In the mid 1990s, the Department of Health gave serious consideration to providing active health and social care support to the public, closer to their own homes. Various initiatives were taken to enhance the care provided in the community. In 1998 the Economics and Operational Research Division of the Department produced a paper making the case that self-care formed a major base of the care pyramid which includes other sectors such as primary, intermediate and hospital care. In 1999 the Government White Paper, *Saving Lives: Our Healthier Nation* specifically recognised that more needed to be done for people with long-term conditions and pointed to the usefulness of self-management training courses.

Towards the end of 1999, the Chief Medical Officer Professor Liam Donaldson set up the Expert Patients Task Force. The Expert Patients Programme emerged from these efforts. The Task Force published its report in September 2001 and the programme began to be rolled out using the generic training method and commissioning the development of disease-specific modules from UK experts.

The generic course uses the reference handbook to accompany the training programme. The handbook consists of chapters which cover issues, problems and their solutions that may be common to a number of chronic disease groups. Common problems may be, among others, fatigue, pain, depression and anxiety. Common solutions may be, among others, relaxation, appropriate diet and exercise. Together these equip participants to build up their confidence in facing life challenges. The handbook covers a number of these topics which are laid out for use in conjunction with the training course.

Disease-specific supplements have been produced and cover conditions such as diabetes, heart disease, asthma, mental illness, irritable bowel syndrome and colitis. Along with the handbook, the supplements will also be made available to the course participants. Where appropriate and necessary, some of the disease-specific training may be delivered in partnership between the professionals and the trained expert patients.

The Expert Patients Programme will ensure equitable provision of self-management training throughout England for people of all ages, gender and ethnicity and covering as many different geographical areas and disease groups as possible.

June 2002

NHS Expert Patients Programme
England

x

How to Become an Expert Patient and Active Self-Manager

THIS HANDBOOK WILL HELP YOU FIND WAYS TO MANAGE YOUR CONDITION AND LEARN A HEALTHY WAY TO LIVE WITH A LONG-TERM OR CHRONIC ILLNESS. This could be heart disease, diabetes, liver disease, depression, asthma, arthritis or any of a host of others. Most of us will have two or more of these conditions during our lives.

You will find out about the common problems people have even if their long-term conditions are different. You will also get plenty of ideas and tips on what to do to deal with your own problems and make your life easier. The advice comes from patients and health / social care professionals. The Expert Patients Programme which provides training in self-management of long-term conditions uses this as a course book. By reading this book along with taking training in self-management of your condition through the Expert Patients Programme you will learn many skills and ways to change your life and become an expert patient.

If you have a chronic condition, you have to choose how you will manage it. You can choose to:

- suffer and do nothing
- just take your medicine
- or take charge and be an active self-manager

Some people manage by staying in bed or withdrawing from life, the disease becomes their centre of focus. Other people with the same condition and symptoms manage to get on with life by changing some of the things they do or the way they get things done. The difference is in how the person decides to live a healthy life with one or more chronic disease(s).

What is a Chronic Condition?

The NHS helps people who have an acute illness such as appendicitis as well as people who have chronic conditions such as arthritis. An acute illness can usually be diagnosed, treated and cured quite quickly. But with the best of intentions chronic diseases often take some time to diagnose and medical or surgical treatment does not lead to a cure.

Various complications can also arise. Some chronic disease can present acutely, such as coronary heart disease. Then there is "acute on chronic disease" which is chronic disease with acute phases. But we may be able to make some general distinction between acute and chronic diseases.

If you have a chronic disease, although doctors can describe the range of symptoms, it may not be possible to tell you exactly what the pattern of your illness will

Table 1.1 *Usual differences between acute and chronic diseases*

	Acute Disease	**Chronic Disease**
Examples	Appendicitis or pneumonia	Arthritis or heart disease
Cause	A single cause such as infection	Many causes such as genetic inheritance, the environment, diet or other lifestyle factors
Diagnosis	Usually easy to diagnose with clear test results	Can be hard to diagnose in the early stages
Duration	Short, over a few days or weeks	Usually lasts for the rest of your life
Effect of Treatment	Can usually be cured with medicine or surgery	Often needs life-long medical treatment and may also need surgery. Symptoms are helped, progress can be slowed but the disease cannot be cured.

be or exactly how the disease will affect you in the future. We do know, however, that people with many different chronic diseases share very similar problems. These common problems include:

- uncertainty
- pain
- tiredness and loss of energy
- poor physical function
- shortness of breath
- worries and depression
- problems with sleeping

The physical problems of chronic conditions can lead to other problems. If you feel tired and have no energy or are in pain or short of breath, you will not want to move around much. This can lead to your muscles becoming weaker and wasted and make it even harder for you to get around. You may then start to feel helpless and start to worry about not getting anything done. When you start to believe that nothing can be done, it becomes very hard to get out of the cycle of helplessness.

Symptoms of chronic conditions can present real challenges. While many people have problems with sleeping, depression can also be a common problem. It is hard to keep cheerful when your disease causes problems that won't go away. You may be worried about the future. 'Will I be able to stay independent?' 'If I can't care for myself, who will care for me?' 'What will happen to my family?'

Through the Expert Patients Programme training course and in this book you will find many ways to help you break the various vicious cycles that you may get into.

Self-Management of Long-Term Condition

No matter what condition you have, you can use your own skills, imagination and information sources to find new approaches to manage your life better. These include:

- learning what to do about day-to-day problems (we could call it problem-solving)
- how to choose an exercise programme
- how to choose a healthy diet
- ways to relax and manage emotions

- ways to manage pain, fatigue or breathing if relevant
- deciding when to seek medical help
- working well with your doctor or other health and social care professionals
- using medicines and reducing side-effects
- finding and using community resources
- talking about your illness to your family and friends

4

The Expert Patients Programme training courses will help you learn these general skills. If you are on an Expert Patients Programme training course, you can also ask for booklets which deal in detail with the causes, problems and treatments of the specific chronic condition or conditions that you have. These booklets may also be available from the local Expert Patients Programme Trainers; ask your Primary Care Trust or call NHS Direct (0845 4647) for their contact details.

A primary problem of living with chronic illness is dealing with this cycle of physical deconditioning and helplessness (see Figure 1.1).

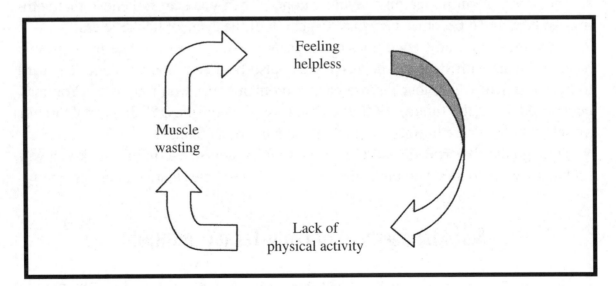

Figure 1.1 *Cycle of helplessness*

The Chronic Illness Path

Understanding and managing your disease means more than learning about the causes and treatment of the condition. It also means finding out how the disease and treatment affect you. With experience, you become the expert in managing life with your condition. BUT self-management does not mean going it alone. The best way to manage a chronic disease is to work in partnership with your doctor or health/social care professional who is caring for you. You will need to tell them how you have been managing and any problems you have had and then discuss whether you need to change your treatment or carry on as before.

Make sure that your doctor tells you which symptoms mean you should seek help urgently. It is important that you tell your doctor about any symptoms which:

- are unusual
- do not go away
- improve, get worse or stay the same
- happen after starting new medicine

5

Most chronic illnesses go up and down in intensity. They do not have a steady path. The visits in Figure 1.2 represent Pat's regular follow-up appointments with a health care professional.

Even though the intensity of Pat's symptoms are at the same level for all three visits, what has happened in between visits needs to be carefully considered. At the first visit symptoms are getting better, at the second visit they are getting worse, and at the third visit things appear to be stable. Treatment will be determined accordingly.

Your experience and understanding of symptoms, communicated clearly to the health professional, would be the best indicators to help determine the right treatment. Skilled health care professionals commonly depend on them. As professionals encourage patients to respond, and patients begin to participate in decisions, a partnership between the two develops. Effective self-management of chronic illness requires such a partnership between patients and care professionals.

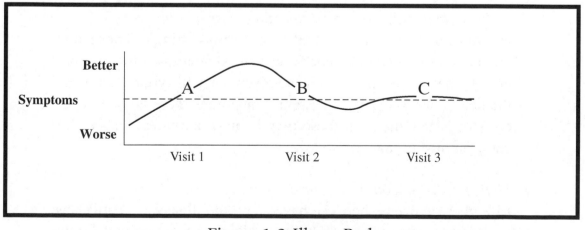

Figure 1.2 *Illness Path*

Table 1.2 *Changes in Pat's Treatment?*

	Symptoms at Visits	Treatment
Visit 1	Getting better	Lessen treatment?
Visit 2	Getting worse	Additional treatment?
Visit 3	Symptoms are stable	Maintain treatment

Self-Management Has to Be Every Day, Not Once in a While

All chronic illnesses need day-to-day management. The extent to which people manage can be different from person to person. But the key to success is:

1. Decide what you want to do.
2. Decide how you are going to do it.
3. Practice regularly what works for you.

What you do about something depends on how you think about it. The thoughts you have can greatly control how you cope with your health related problems.

Some of the best self-managers think of their illness as a path. The path goes up and down, sometimes it is flat and smooth, and at other times it is rough. Sometimes you can get things done quickly, and other times you must slow down; there may be obstacles and you have to find ways and means to get through them. The best self-managers learn the skills they need to travel on the path. These are:

- *Skills to deal with the illness and manage symptoms*
  Having an illness means that you do new things. These may include taking medicine, checking your symptoms, or using oxygen. It means you have more involvement with your doctor and the health and social care system. Sometimes there are new exercises or a new diet. All these may be new activities you need to carry out just to manage your illness.

- *Skills needed to continue your normal life*
  Life goes on even when you have a chronic illness. You still have housework, friendships to keep up, jobs to manage and family

relationships to keep going. Things that you once took for granted can become much more complicated. You may need to learn new ways to do old things and enjoy life.

- *Skills needed to deal with emotions*
When you are diagnosed as having a chronic illness, your future plans may have to change and changes can lead to negative emotions. They may include: anger —'Why me? It's not fair'; depression — 'I can't do anything any more, what's the use'; frustration — 'No matter what I do it doesn't make any difference'; or isolation — 'No one understands, no one wants to be around someone who is ill.' **BUT** you can learn how to deal with these negative emotions. The Expert Patients Programme training course will help you do just that.

7

Self-management is using skills you have learnt to:

    1. deal with your illness and manage your symptoms;

    2. continue your daily activities; and

    3. manage your emotions.

How to Become a Day-to-Day Active Self-Manager

Like any skill, active self-management can be learned and practised. Remember: **You are the manager**; so to take charge you must take seven steps :

    1. Decide what you want to achieve.
    2. Look for different ways to achieve this goal.
    3. Start making short-term plans by making an action plan.
    4. Carry out your action plans.
    5. Check the results.
    6. Make changes as needed.
    7. Remember to reward yourself.

Problems sometimes start by you feeling a bit uneasy. Let's say you are unhappy but not sure why. By thinking about it more, you find you miss contact with an old friend who has moved. You decide to go and visit this friend. You now know your goal. The following chart shows the steps to achieving your goal.

Planning a visit to a friend

Step	Choices	Information Needed	Problem	Decision
How to get there	A. Drive myself	Road map and mileage	Too tiring	Go for Choice B
	B. Take a coach	Coach timetables	Coach station too far from friend's house	Go for Choice C
	C. Go by train	Train timetables	Getting to and from station	Decide to go by train and take a bus or ask a neighbour for a ride to the station
When to travel	During daylight but off-peak hours	Off-peak fares	None likely	Avoid rush hours and crowding and unnecessary expense
Luggage	Use old suitcase		Hard to carry	
	Buy new case with wheels	Cost		Decide to use old case and ask for porter to help get on & off the train

8

Make an *action plan* and *carry it out*

- Phone or visit your local station to find out what help they can offer people with poor mobility.
- Take a short walk each day to get steadier on your feet.
- Walk up and down steps with bag to get more confident.

Check the results

- The train staff were very helpful and reduced your worries about the journey.

- Your walking is not as good as you'd hoped, so you decide to ask a physiotherapist for help. She suggests using a stick, which you hate but try and find that it does help and gives extra support on a moving train.

The Seven Self-Management Steps in More Detail

1. Deciding what you want to achieve

Deciding on your goal may be difficult. You must be realistic and very specific. Think of all the things you would like to do. One example is of someone who wanted to climb twenty steps to her daughter's home so that she could join her family for a special meal. Another person wanted to lose weight to help his cardiac condition. Someone else wanted to get out and do more but felt limited by having to take her oxygen tank everywhere. Each of these goals will take several weeks or months to achieve.

There may be times when you are uncertain about what may be considered a realistic goal, for example, to decide how many steps to climb. In such a situation you will need to set a goal in partnership with your doctor or other health / social care professionals.

One of the problems with goals is that they may often seem like dreams, so unlikely that we don't even try to tackle them. Write down your goals and decide which one you want to work on first.

Goals:

1st) _____

2nd) _____

3rd) _____

2. Looking for different ways to achieve your goal

Sometimes, what stops us reaching our goal is not seeing or thinking about the other ways it could be done. There are many ways to reach any goal. For example, the mother who wanted to climb 20 steps could start off with a slow walking programme; climb up and down a few steps each day; or she could look into having the special family meal at a different place. The man who wanted to lose weight could decide not to eat between meals; give up desserts; or start an exercise programme. The woman who wanted to do more could find out about courses at a local Further Education College; join an Expert Patient Programme; or phone or write letters to friends.

Your job is to list all the ways you can think of and then choose one or two to work with that appeal to you. If you are having problems thinking of different choices, then ask your family, friends or care professionals for their suggestions. You could also try asking other people in your community such as work colleagues or local club, charity or religious leaders.

Don't assume that a choice does not exist or will not work until you have properly looked into it. There is always more going on in your community than you might expect. For example, a woman who had lived in the same town her whole life was having trouble arranging for hospital transport to take her to her appointments and a friend suggested a voluntary car scheme. However, the woman thought that this service did not exist in her town. It was only when her friend came to visit several months later and called a local voluntary agency that she learnt the town had three voluntary schemes and one Council run service that could help her. So, never assume anything.

Write down a list of different ways to reach your top goal. Decide which two or three you would like to try.

Choices

1st) _____

2nd) _____

3rd) _____

4th) _____

3. Making Short-Term Plans: Action Planning

Now you need to turn your choices into short-term plans: an action plan. This is a set of actions you know you will be able to take in the next week. The action plan should be about something you want to get done; it is not to please your family or doctor.

Action plans are a very important self-management tool. We all know we can do things to make us healthier, but we fail to do them. For example, most people with a chronic illness can walk, some just across the room, others can walk a mile or so. BUT few people have a proper exercise programme.

How to make an action plan

i. *Decide what you will do this week.* A step-climber might decide to climb three steps once a day for four days. A man trying to lose weight may decide not to eat between meals for three days and to walk round the block before dinner on the following four days. The action must be something you can do. If in doubt, you may want to work in partnership with health and social care professionals.

ii. *Make sure your plans link to an exact behaviour.* Rather than decide just 'to relax'; decide, 'I will listen to my progressive muscle relaxation tape.'

iii. *Make a detailed plan.* The plan should consist of all the following steps:
    a. *Exactly **what** are you going to do?* How far will you walk? How will you eat less? What breathing technique will you practise?
    b. *How **much** will you do?* Will you walk for 15 minutes? Not ea t between meals for three days? Practise breathing exercises for 15 minutes?
    c. ***When** will you do this?* Before lunch? When I come home from work? Connecting a new activity to an old habit is a good way to make sure it gets done. Another trick is to do your new activity before a favourite activity such as reading the newspaper.
    d. *How **often** will you do the activity?* It is not always possible to do things every day, it is best to decide to do things three, four or five times a week. You will feel less pressure and be more likely to succeed with your action plan. (Please note: Taking medicines must be done exactly as directed by your doctor or pharmacist).

e. *Start where you are or start **slowly***. If you wish to start increasing your physical activity then there is useful advice in chapter 4. If you are in doubt about starting even very slowly on walking and exercise, you should take a decision in partnership with your health and social care professionals.

iv. *Give yourself some time off.*

v. *Ask yourself how confident you are.* 'On a scale of 0 to 10, with 0 being totally unsure and 10 being totally certain, answer *how confident am I* that I can complete this plan?' If you answer 7 or over, your plan will probably work. If you answer below 7, look at your plan again and ask yourself what problems you think there will be. See if you can solve the problems or change your plan to make yourself more certain you will succeed.

vi. *Write down your plan.* Put it where you will see it easily every day. Make a regular note of any problems you have. (There is an example of an action plan at the end of this chapter.)

A Successful Action Plan must be:

1. Something YOU want to do
2. Reasonable (something you have thought through thoroughly and feel you will be able to achieve)
3. Linked to a specific behaviour (e.g. not eating after dinner)
4. Detailed and must answer the questions:
   i. What?
   ii. How much?
   iii. When?
   iv. How often?
5. Confidence level of 7 or more (something you are very confident you can do)

4. Carrying Out Your Action Plan

A well thought-out plan is easy to follow. Ask your family or friends to check on how you are doing; telling them about your progress will keep you motivated. Tick things off on your chart when you finish doing them. Make notes of any problems you have. The notes will help you see if there is a pattern to any problems.

5. Check Your Results

At the end of each week, see how much of your action plan you have carried out. Think about how near you are to reaching your goal. You should see a little progress each week. If you are having problems, you need to solve them.

6. Make Changes

Early on if there are difficulties, don't give up, try something else. Change your short-term plans so that your steps are easier, give yourself more time, get more advice or help from other people, especially your fellow self-managers.

- Work out what the real problem is. For example: you know the stairs are a problem, but it takes a bit more thought to work out that your real problem is a fear of falling.

- Make a list of ideas to solve the problem. You can ask other people to help you with this.

- Pick one idea to try. Remember that new activities are often difficult.

- Think about how you have done when you've given your idea a chance to work.

- If you still have the problem, try another of your ideas or ask other people for their advice.

If you can find no way to solve your problem, you will have to accept that you may not be able to solve your problem now. You can try later or you can think about other ways to reach your goal.

> ## Summary of problem-solving steps
>
> 1. **Identify the problem.**
> 2. **List ideas to solve the problem.**
> 3. **Select one method to try.**
> 4. **Think about the results.**
> 5. **Try another idea if the first didn't work.**
> 6. **Use other resources (ask friends, family or professionals for ideas)**
> 7. **Accept that the problem may not be solvable now.**

14

7. Rewards of Being a Self-Manager

The best part of being a good self-manager is the reward you get when you achieve your goals and live a fuller and more comfortable life. Set simple and easy goals and you will reward yourself often. For example:

- Decide you won't read the paper until after your exercise; reading the paper becomes your reward.

- Stop smoking and use the money saved to buy fruits instead, or have an outing with the family or a friend.

Rewards don't have to be expensive or fattening! There are many healthy pleasures that can add enjoyment to your life.

Please remember that not all goals are achievable. Chronic illness may mean having to give some things up. Don't think too much about what you can't do, but start to work on a goal you can achieve. Talk about all the things you can do.

This handbook provides resource material to support the training you are undergoing in self-management of your life with long-term condition(s). It will also be a good reminder of the lessons you would learn at the training. The first and last chapters may be worth going through fully. You can skip around the other chapters or the disease-specific supplements depending on the information you are looking for. The table of contents at the beginning or the index at the back may prove to be a valuable guide.

Example of an Action Plan

When you write your action plan, be sure it includes:

1. what you are going to do
2. how much you are going to do
3. when you are going to do it
4. how many days a week you are going to do it

For example:

This week ......
what: I will walk around the block
how much: twice
when: before lunch
how many: three days this week.

How confident are you that you can complete this plan?
(0= not at all confident; 10= totally confident)
Record your score here: _____9_____

Record your comments on how your plan went

	Tick	Comments
Monday	—	*Raining*
Tuesday	✓	*Walked slowly & noticed everything around me*
Wednesday	✓	*It was cool out, but the walk felt good*
Thursday	—	*Raining again*
Friday	✓	*Only walked around the block once*
Saturday	✓	*Took a friend along, we talked about the neighbours*
Sunday	—	*Felt tired*
Overall Comment		*Exceeded my expectations and walked around the block four days this week.*

Action Plan Form

When you write your action plan, be sure it includes:

1. what you are going to do
2. how much you are going to do
3. when you are going to do it
4. how many days a week you are going to do it

16

[For example, I will walk around the block (*what*) twice (*how much*) before lunch (*when*) three days this week (*how many*).]

My Action Plan this week:

what: _____

how much: _____

when: _____

how many days: _____

How confident are you that you can complete this plan?
(0= not at all confident; 10= totally confident)

Record your comments on how your plan went

	Tick	Comments
Monday		
Tuesday		
Wednesday		
Thursday		
Friday		
Saturday		
Sunday		
Overall Comment		

• • •

Suggested Further Reading

Cousins, Norman. *Anatomy of an Illness as Perceived by the Patient: Reflections on Healing and Regeneration.* New York: W.W. Norton and Co., 1995.

Klein, Robert A., and Marcia Goodman Landau. *Healing: The Body Betrayed.* Minneapolis, Minn.: DCI Publishing, 1992. (Self-paced, self-help guide to regaining psychological control of your chronic illness.)

Lorig, Kate and James Fries. *The Arthritis Self Help Book.* 5th Edition, Addison-Wesley, 2001.

Milstrey Wells, S. *A Delicate Balance: Living Successfully with Chronic Illness.* Perseus Books Group, 2000.

Sobel, David and Robert Ornstein. *Healthy Pleasures.* 2nd ed. Mass: Addison-Wesley, 1997.

CHAPTER
2
Finding Resources

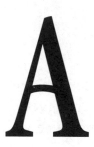 MAJOR PART OF BECOMING A SELF-MANAGER OF YOUR CHRONIC ILL-
NESS IS KNOWING WHEN YOU NEED HELP AND HOW YOU CAN FIND
HELP.

Your family or friends may be your first source of help. In the chapter on *Communicating* there is advice on how to choose the right words to ask for help. Some people find it hard to ask for help from people they know and some people do not have family or friends they can call on. There are other resources in your community you can look for.

Finding what you need may be as simple as looking in the telephone book and making some phone calls or it may take more effort and thought.

For example, you are finding it difficult to prepare meals because you can't stand up for very long. But you want to keep on cooking for yourself. You decide to get your kitchen altered so you can prepare meals sitting down.

You start by talking to other people who can give you leads; they may remember someone who has had similar work done. You could find out a lot about costs and problems from them.

You might look in the yellow pages for builders or architects. Some of them specialise in kitchens, but none mention anything about designing for people with physical limitations. After a couple of phone calls you can't find anyone with the right experience in design.

Who else could you try? You could look for names in the local paper or see if anyone has advertised their details at the local post office or the corner shop. Perhaps contact the Occupational Therapist in your local social services department? Explore the databases in your library reference section? The Citizens'

Advice Bureau has a resource database. You could also seek support at your regular place of worship.

There are some people in every community who seem to know who is who and where everything is. They tend to be people who have been living there a long time and who have got involved in the community. These people are **natural** problem solvers. You may know someone like this "Natural" who would know the answer or who could set you on the right path to finding the answer. Sometimes the "Natural" is a friend, a person who runs a local club, a religious leader of any faith, a doctor or school secretary, a librarian, the postman, or someone who works at the local newsagents. All you do is think of this person as an information source. Once you get good at thinking about and using your community resources, you will soon find that other people start to use you as their "Natural" information source.

Resources for Resources

When we need to find goods or services, there are certain resources we can call on in order to find more resources. The "Natural" is one of those resources, but we need a variety of other tools to be fully successful in finding the service we are looking for.

Some examples are:

- The telephone directory — the business pages of the local BT Phonebook, Yellow Pages or the Thompson Directory

- Your local library

- Disabled Living Centre or Independent Living Centre; they keep up-to-date catalogues of equipment for people with any form of physical problem

- Shops and Pharmacies supplying medical equipment

- Council for Voluntary Service or Rural Community Council

- National Council for Voluntary Organisations

- Voluntary groups dedicated to your disease; if you can't find a local branch, you will need to find their national office

- There are a large number of telephone helpline services now available; a full list is kept by the College of Health in London;

also the local library will be able to get you this list.; health and social care related voluntary agencies dedicated to a disease may have a helpline, such as Arthritis Care, BACUP (cancer), Diabetes UK, the National Asthma Campaign, the British Heart Foundation, or the Multiple Sclerosis Society

- The BBC has helplines and services that can be contacted after certain programmes

The patient support organisations provide up-to-date information about your disease and advice, plus guidance and support on daily living issues. Many of them fund research that they hope will help people live better with their disease and may lead to a cure. They will send you newsletters and information leaflets on request; for a membership fee, you can also join these organisations.

Most patient support organisations have good Internet websites. You can also find out how people with your condition get help anywhere in the world.

Financial Matters

Citizens' Advice Bureaus, Law Centres and Independent Welfare Rights groups (usually affiliated to the Federation of Independent Advice Centres FIAC) are good places to visit to find out about state benefits or financial matters. Some Social Services Departments in cities also offer these services. Some will make home visits to help you sort out problems. Benefits Plus (which used to be called the Benefits Agency) does not have to advise you in your best interests, it only has to provide you accurate information. It is a good idea to use independent agencies to get a full review of the benefits you are entitled to.

Other Organisations

There are other types of organisations from where you may be able to get help. Some of these are:

- *Ex-military organisations* if you or a close relative have been in the forces. The Royal British Legion or the Soldiers, Sailors and Airman's Families Association (SSAFA) can give you information.

- *Religious organisations.* Many religious organisations have advisory services. You do not need to be a member of a religious organisation to receive help. Local Parishes, Diocese, The Salvation Army, Mosques, Temples or Gurdwaras, for example, have good information about local services.

- *Domestic violence organisations.* Domestic violence against people with chronic disease can happen. Local refuges treat all enquiries seriously and in confidence. Their addresses are not made public but they can be contacted through the local police or social services.

22

- *Local authority services.* Housing Advice Centres can help you find somewhere to live or find grants to improve things such as heating and insulation. Social services have a duty to provide advice for disabled people. The advice is free, but you have to buy, or contribute towards, any equipment you may need. There may be grants that you can apply for if you do not have adequate resources.

- *Disability Employment Advisors (DEA)* are attached to Job Centres run by the employment agency. They can help you if you are working and have a chronic disease or disability that will last for more than six months. They can also help if you are planning to get back to work. The Disability Discrimination Act gives you real protection and can help to make sure your employer is able to find ways to keep you employed by providing special equipment or facilities. Do not think about quitting a job on the grounds of ill health until you have talked to a DEA.

- *NHS Direct* is a telephone and website service run mainly by nurses who can give health-related information. They can give you advice over the phone (0845 4647) or can suggest what you should do next.

- *Local Librarians* can help you use the computer databases and reference section of a library. Make sure that any medical or health-related books you use to get information have been published very recently as a specific treatment may have changed. Librarians will know about specialist libraries not open to the public and can order books and journals for you from anywhere in the country. For a small fee, you can order copies of articles published in journals. You may be able to get access to a university medical library which will have a wide collection of books and journals. Medical books may contain information in great detail. Use the information of interest or relevance to you. You may find details about helpful organisations at the back of books, and there will also be reading lists and bibliographies at the end for more sources of information.

- *Government documents* can be bought through HMSO (Her Majesty's Stationery Office) or they can be downloaded from government websites for free.

23

- *Local and national newspapers* sometimes have a health editor who may have a file of information or may even be interested in helping you to track down something you want to read. In relevant sections of newspapers, local organisations advertise classes, lectures and meetings that you could attend.

The Internet and the World Wide Web

The Internet is the fastest growing resource in the world. It is a great information source and it allows you to interact with people all over the world. If you have a rare medical disease, you can find other people with the same condition to chat with.

BUT, anyone can post any information they like on a Website. There are very few controls. Do not assume that any information on the Internet is true. You need to think about the following points:

- Is the author or sponsor of the Website clearly identified?
- Is the author reputable?
- Are they trying to sell you something?

Study the Website address, the URL (Uniform Resource Locator), which starts with http://. For example, the Department of Health website is: http://www.doh.gov.uk/

http:// means 'hyper text transfer protocol.' 'www' means that the website is on the World Wide Web. 'doh' is short for Department of Health. 'gov' means that the website is a government site. 'uk' means that the site has originated in the UK.

You will often see .edu, .org, .gov or .com as part of a website's URL. If there are no initials for a country (such as uk) at the end of a URL, it means the website is probably based in the USA.

In the UK, URLs ending with .ac.uk indicate that it is an academic institution.

Private, voluntary organisations and 'not-for-profit' organisations have .org.uk at the end. Private companies in the UK also may have .co.uk at the end.

If you want to try using the web for the first time, many libraries now have computers which you can use for a small fee or you could try an Internet Café. If you think you might use the Internet a great deal on your home computer, look out for special Internet connection packages to avoid huge telephone bills.

Here are some examples of useful health-related websites in the UK

24

NHS Direct
www.nhsdirect.nhs.uk

Access to Care Website provides an understanding about the issues affecting access to health care services in the UK
http://www.his.path.cam.ac.uk/phealth/access/access.htm

BBC health
http://www.bbc.co.uk/health/

What should I do? describes a number of commonly occurring health problems and provides advice about what you can do yourself
http://www.whatshouldido.com/

DIPEx is the world's first Database of Individual Patient Experiences in Hypertension, Prostate and Breast Cancer
http://www.dipex.org/

British Medical Journal
http://www.bmj.com/index.shtml

Information on BSE
http://www.cjd.ed.ac.uk

OMNI (Organizing Medical Networked Information) is a gateway to Internet resources in medicine, and health care
http://omni.nott.ac.uk

The Long Term Medical Conditions Alliance's website provides specific information about the Chronic Disease Self-Management Course, and useful contacts:
www.lmca.org.uk

Public Health Genetics Unit provides news and information about advances in genetics and their impact on prevention of disease
http://www.medinfo.cam.ac.uk/phgu/default.asp

Disabled Living Foundation
www.dlf.org.uk

Patient UK is a directory of health, disease and related websites from the UK
www.patient.co.uk

25

Age Concern
www.ageconcern.org.uk

Arthritis Care
www.arthritiscare.org.uk

British Heart Foundation
www.bhf.org.uk

Diabetes UK
www.diabetes.org.uk

Multiple Sclerosis Society
www.mssociety.org.uk

National Asthma Campaign
www.asthma.org.uk

Femail netdoctor has good information on medicines; it is the medical section of the Daily Mail's women's section
http://femail.netdoctor.co.uk

Some useful USA and Canadian sites

About.com provides links to a network of Alternative Medicine sites
http://www.altmedicine.about.com/health/altmedicine/

Centers for Disease Prevention and Control
www.cdc.gov/

Dr Koop Website provides information on 60 different health conditions such as HIV/AIDS, depression, allergies, diabetes, Alzheimer's, heart disease, arthritis, hypertension, asthma, mental health, cancer, migraine etc.
http://www.drkoop.com/

Health AtoZ
www.healthatoz.com/

HealthGrades provides US ratings of hospitals, doctors and Health plans to help people select the best quality providers of medical care
http://www.healthgrades.com

Healthwise handbooks provide self-care guide for 180 common health problems
http://www.healthwise.org/

InteliHealth is a leading online health information company from sources such as Harvard Medical School
http://www.intelihealth.com/

Johns Hopkins University Health Information
www.intelihealth.com/IH/ihtIH

Mayo Clinic
www.mayohealth.org/

Medical Matrix is a free directory of selected medical sites on the Internet; it lists only those sites that meet criteria for information quality, with an emphasis on usefulness to healthcare practitioners
http://www.medmatrix.org/

Medscape offers useful medical information and educational programs on the Internet
http://www.medscape.com/

Medicinal herbs provides answers to frequently asked questions associated to herbal medicine
http://www.ibiblio.org/herbmed/index.html

Internet Mental Health is a free encyclopedia of mental health information
http://www.mentalhealth.com

National Institutes of Health
www.nih.gov/

National Library of Medicine, PubMed and MedLine, USA
http://www.nlm.nih.gov/

Nutritional Supplements has information about nutritional supplements and pre-scription drugs
http://www.nutritionalsupplements.com

Nursing Site — Worldwide Nurse
http://www.wwnurse.com

OnLine Surgery to view general procedures as well as cosmetic procedures
http://www.onlinesurgery.com

PubMed is a US National Library of Medicine's on-line search service
http://www.ncbi.nlm.nih.gov/PubMed

Self Care website looking at such topics as fitness, nutrition, pregnancy etc.
http://www.phys.com

Tufts University Nutrition Navigator
http://navigator.tufts.edu/

The Virtual Hospital digital library contains hundreds of books and brochures on health information for doctors and patients
http://www.vh.org

Web MD provides high-quality health care information on a number of diseases and health related topics
http://www.webmd.com

Yoga Studio takes people through a yoga class
http://www.timages.com/yoga.htm

CHAPTER 3

Taking Control by Managing Symptoms

Understanding Common Symptoms

IN THIS CHAPTER, YOU WILL LEARN HOW TO MANAGE THE COMMON SYMP-TOMS OF CHRONIC ILLNESS. The symptoms of chronic illnesses are signals from the body that something is happening. The symptoms are hard to describe and you can't predict when they are going to happen. They will affect you in a very personal way. The common symptoms of chronic illness include:

- Fatigue
- Stress
- Shortness of breath
- Pain
- Itching
- Anger
- Depression
- Sleep problems

You can have several of the symptoms at the same time and some symptoms can make others worse or lead to new problems.

Learning to manage symptoms is very similar to problem solving (see Chapter 1). There are steps you can follow to help you manage the symptoms. First you need to identify which symptom you have; then you need to work out what is causing the symptom. Each symptom may have many causes and the symptoms can affect your life in different ways.

Many symptoms have the same causes. As you learn more about the causes, you may find ways to prevent certain symptoms from coming back.

Fatigue

Having a chronic illness can drain your energy and fatigue is a real problem and not "all in the mind". Unfortunately, other people sometimes do not understand how fatigue can just suddenly hit you. They may think you are just not interested or want to be alone.

There may be many reasons for your fatigue such as:

- **The disease itself.** To do anything, you need energy. When you have a chronic illness, your body needs energy to repair the damage caused by your illness. This means you may not have enough energy left for everyday activities.

- **Not being active.** When you don't use muscles, they become wasted and don't work well. The heart is made of muscle and it can also become less efficient. This means the heart will not be good at pumping blood, nutrients and oxygen around the body. When muscles do not get food and oxygen, they cannot work properly. Muscles that are wasted get tired more easily than muscles that are in good condition. Believing you can't exercise because you are too tired leads to a vicious circle. People get into a state of always feeling tired because they do not exercise enough. If this is your problem, you need to start a gentle exercise programme. Chapter 4 will give you more information on how to do this.

- **Poor diet.** Food is our basic source of energy. If you eat poor food or don't eat the right amount of food, you can get fatigued more easily. If you are eating too much junk food or drinking too much alcohol, then you need to eat better quality food in the proper quantities. If you can't eat much and are losing weight, you need to think carefully about the type of food you eat. Chapter 10 gives more details about food and eating habits.

- **Weight problems.** For some people, being obese can lead to fatigue. Extra weight causes an increase in the amount of energy you need to do anything. For other people, being underweight can cause fatigue.

- **Emotions.** Feeling under stress can lead to fatigue. Fatigue is a major symptom of depression.

- **Not enough sleep.** Not enough sleep or poor quality sleep can result in fatigue.

Stress

Stress is a common problem for everybody. Your body is used to working at a certain level. When you have to do something extra, your body prepares for physical action and makes sure oxygen and energy are sent to your muscles. This causes your heart rate to increase, your blood pressure rises, your breathing becomes more rapid, your neck and shoulder muscles tense, your mouth becomes dry and you may begin sweating. These are the body's response to stress and usually only last until the stressful event is over. If the stress is present for a long time, the body begins to adapt to the stress. This can lead or add to other problems such as hypertension, shortness of breath or muscle and joint pain.

Common Types of Stressors

Stressors are activities, incidents, feelings or things that causes stress. Let us look at a few examples of stressors.

- *Physical stressors.* These increase your body's demand for energy. A physical stressor can be something pleasant like picking up your grandchild or it could be a big shopping trip demanding a lot of energy. The physical symptoms of your illness can cause stress. If your body is not able to deal with the demand for energy, you may get sore muscles or even a worsening of disease symptoms.

- *Chemical stressors.* Cigarettes, coffee, alcohol or drugs can act as chemical stressors.

- *Mental and emotional stressors.* These can range from pleasant to uncomfortable feelings. Joyful experiences such as family weddings lead to the same stress response in your body as feeling frustrated or down because of your illness.

- *Environmental stressors.* These can also be good or bad and include things like a sunny day, uneven pavements that make it difficult to walk, loud noises, or smoky rooms.

31

Good Stress

Exercise is another example of a good stress that puts demands on your body. Your heart has to work harder to get blood to the muscles, your lungs have to work harder and you breathe more quickly to keep up with your muscles' need for oxygen. Your muscles are working hard to keep up with signals from your brain telling them to keep moving.

If you keep on with an exercise programme for several weeks, you will begin to see changes. What seemed nearly impossible at the start will get much easier. Your body will adapt to the stress. There will be less strain on your heart, lungs and muscles which will become more efficient and you will become more fit.

32

How to Recognise When You Feel Stressed

Stress is helpful as long as you do not go past the 'breaking point' when your life starts to feel out of control. It can be hard to know when you are getting to this point, some of the signs include:

- Biting your nails, pulling your hair
- Grinding your teeth, clenching your jaw
- Tensing your head, neck or shoulders
- Feeling anxious, nervous, helpless or irritable
- Having many accidents or forgetting things you don't normally forget

You can sometimes catch yourself doing these things or feeling in these ways. If you think you are feeling this way, take a few minutes to think about what it is that is making you feel tense. Take a few deep breaths and try to relax. There are some relaxation methods later on in this chapter.

How to Deal with Stress

- **Avoiding stressful situations.** There are some situations you know will always be stressful such as going on a long journey or preparing a meal. First you need to work out what it is about the situation that you find stressful. Is it that you hate to be late? Do you worry about parking? Does cooking demand too much energy? Then begin to look for possible ways to reduce the stress. Can you leave earlier? Can you use public transport? Can you prepare the meal in stages? Choose one solution and try it next time you are in this kind of situation.

- **Managing the stress.** Develop ways to deal with the stressful situations before they happen. Go over in your head what you will do in that situation. You need to listen to and recognise your body's signals that stress is building up. Nicotine, alcohol and caffeine can increase stress. Some people smoke a cigarette, drink a glass of wine or drink a cup of coffee to soothe tension, but these actions actually increase the body's stress response. Try to cut down on these chemical stressors. Other ways to deal with stress include:
  — Self-talk, progressive muscle relaxation and guided imagery
  — Getting enough sleep or getting treatment for a sleep disorder, if appropriate
  — Exercising
  — Eating well

Shortness of Breath

If you have shortness of breath, it means your body is not getting the oxygen it needs. Chronic illness can lead to changes in the body which can make you become short of breath.

Causes of Shortness of Breath

- *Damage to the air sacs in the lungs.* This means the lungs can't get enough oxygen into the blood and carbon dioxide out of the blood.

- *Narrowing of the airways to the air sacs and production of too much mucus.* Less air can flow through the narrow airways to the lungs.

- *The heart not pumping blood efficiently.* The heart can't work hard enough to meet the body's oxygen needs leaving you feeling short of breath as your breathing speeds up to try to meet the need for oxygen.

- *Being overweight.* Added weight increases the amount of energy and oxygen the body needs to do anything. This means the heart has to work harder.

- *Wasting of muscles.* Muscle wasting can affect the breathing muscles. Wasted muscles become less efficient and need more energy and oxygen, clearing air in and out of the lungs becomes less efficient.

Shortness of Breath is Frightening and Fear Can Lead To:

1. A release of hormones that cause more shortness of breath.

2. You stopping what you are doing. This means that you will not build up the endurance to exercise that you need to help your breathing.

How to Manage Shortness of Breath

> When you feel short of breath, *don't stop what you are doing or hurry up to finish, but slow down.* If shortness of breath carries on, then stop for a few minutes. Take any medicine that has been prescribed by your doctor.

1. *Take things slowly and in steps.*

2. *Increase your level of activity slowly each week.* For example, if you are able to work in the garden for 20 minutes, increase it by no more than five minutes the next week. Once you can work comfortably for 25 minutes, you can add a few more minutes.

3. *Don't smoke and avoid smokers.* This may be difficult if you have friends or family who smoke. You need to explain that their smoking is causing you to have problems in breathing. Ask people to smoke outside.

4. *Use your medicines and oxygen.* Medicines can be lifesavers if you have a chronic disease. Don't try to cut down or go without the medication and don't take more than you are prescribed. You may have to take medicines even when you have no symptoms. If you feel your medicine is not working, talk to your doctor before you stop taking the medicine or change the dose.

5. *Drink plenty of fluids (unless your doctor has advised you to restrict your fluids).* This is helpful if mucus and secretions are a problem for you as it will thin the mucus and make it easier to cough up. A humidifier may also help.

6. *Practise pursed-lip and diaphragmatic breathing.* This can help strengthen and improve your breathing muscles as well as reduce the amount of energy you need to breathe. You can use these methods to help you relax.

Pursed-lip breathing

- *Breathe in through your nose.* (This may be easier if you lean forward.)

- *Hold your breath briefly.*

- *With your lips pursed* (as if you were going to whistle), *breathe out slowly through your lips.* Breathing out should take twice as long as breathing in.

- *Practise* this technique for five to ten minutes, two to four times a day.

Diaphragmatic breathing

- *Lie on your back* with pillows under your head and knees.

- *Place one hand on your stomach* (at the base of your breastbone) and the other hand on your upper chest.

- *Breathe in slowly through your nose,* allowing your stomach to expand outward. Imagine that your lungs are getting filled with fresh air. The hand on your stomach should move upward, and the hand on your chest should not move or only move slightly.

- *Breathe out slowly, through pursed lips.* At the same time, use your hand to gently push inward and upward on your abdomen.

- *Practise* this technique for ten to fifteen minutes, three or four times a day, until it becomes automatic. If you begin to feel a little dizzy, then you must rest.

35

When you are comfortable doing this, you can place a light weight on your abdomen. This will help to strengthen the muscles you use to breathe in. Start with a weight of about one pound (500 grams) like a book or a bag of rice or beans. Over the weeks, increase the weight as your muscle strength improves. After you can breathe easily lying down, you can practise diaphragmatic breathing while you are sitting, standing and finally, while walking. When you can master this method while you are doing other activities, you will be better able to manage your shortness of breath.[1]

36

Pain

For many people with chronic illness, pain and physical discomfort are their main problems. The five most common causes are:

- *The disease itself.* Pain can be due to inflammation, damage in or around joints and tissues, lack of proper blood supply to the heart, damage to the nervous system or trapped nerves.

- *Tense muscles.* When something hurts, the muscles in that area become tense. This is a natural reaction to pain, to try to protect the area that is damaged. When muscles are tensed for a long time, lactic acid builds up in the muscles which can also cause pain.

- *Muscle wasting.* When a muscle is weak, it feels sore and painful any time it is used. Even the slightest activity can sometimes lead to pain and stiffness.

- *Lack of good quality sleep.* Pain can stop you either getting to sleep or having a good sleep. This can make pain worse and leave you less able to cope with it.

- *Emotions and stress.* Anxiety, depression, anger, fear and frustration can affect the way you feel pain, making it seem worse.

Managing Pain

- *Medicines.* Some medicines can help. For example, those that open blood vessels and bronchial tubes and those that reduce

---

[1] The material on pursed-lip, diaphragmatic and pursed-lip breathing was taken from the following two publications: *Essentials of Pulmonary Rehabilitation* by Thomas L. Petty, M.D., Brian Tiep, M.D., and Mary Burns, R.N., B.S. Pulmonary Education and Research Foundation, P.O. Box 1133, Lomita, CA 90717-5133; and *Help Yourself to Better Breathing*, American Lung Association, 1989.

inflammation. Painkillers such as narcotics are **not** helpful for chronic diseases. Narcotics can be dangerous for people who have damaged lungs as they slow down the breathing rate and can make existing breathing problems worse. Painkillers can become less effective over time and some are addictive.

- *Exercise, and techniques where you use your mind such as relaxation and visualisation.* These are good ways to deal with pain and are discussed later in this chapter.

- *Use of heat.* Heat can stimulate the skin around the painful area and improve the blood supply. Use a heating pad or take a bath or shower and direct the flow of hot water at the area. Make a heating pad by filling a sock with rice or dry beans, knotting the top and putting it in a microwave oven for three to four minutes. Test the heat before you use it so as not to burn yourself.

- *Use of cold.* A cold pack can be helpful if pain is caused by inflammation for example in MS or rheumatoid arthritis. Use a bag of frozen peas.

- *Massage.* Self-massage stimulates the skin, tissues and muscles by applying pressure. You can use a mentholated cream if you want a cooling effect. **Do not** use massage for a hot joint (one that is red, swollen and hot to the touch) or an infected area or if you have phlebitis, thrombophlebitis or skin eruptions.

- *Pain-management clinic.* You can ask to be referred to a pain-management clinic if you cannot find a way to manage your pain.

Itching

Itching is any sensation that causes an urge to scratch. There are many causes. People with liver disease may have itching caused by bile products deposited in the skin. Kidney disease may lead to itching but we do not know why. The skin condition psoriasis also leads to severe problems with itching.

Managing and Relieving Itching

If your itching is caused by histamines released by an allergic reaction or through contact with an irritating substance, you must wash off the substance, apply a cold compress and take an antihistamine medicine, such as diphenhydramine (Benadryl).

37

- *Moisture.* Dry skin is itchy, so use a moisturising cream several times a day. Read the list of ingredients before you buy a product and avoid ones which contain alcohol or any ingredient that ends in "ol" as they tend to dry the skin. The greasier the product, the better it works as a moisturiser. You can buy 'Emulsifying Ointment' from a pharmacy; it works well and is cheap. Use warm water in baths or showers and soak for not less than 10 and not more than 20 minutes. You can try adding home-made bath oil made from 2 teaspoons of olive oil and a large glass of milk. When you get out of the water, pat yourself dry and apply your cream. In cold weather, indoor heating dries the skin; a humidifier can help or you can keep your home and office as cool as possible.

- *Clothing.* Clothes made from natural fibres such as cotton allow the skin to 'breathe' more easily and are least irritating.

- *Medicines.* Antihistamines help if your itching is caused by the release of histamines. You can buy these over-the-counter: triprolidine (Actifed), diphenhydramine (Benadryl), and chlorpheniramine (Calimal, Piriton). Some creams help to soothe the nerve endings such as Algipam and Vicks VapoRub. Anti-itch creams contain benzocaine, lidocaine or pramoxine. Capsaicin creams help itching but cause a burning sensation. Steroid creams control some types of itching. Consult your doctor or the pharmacist if you need to use these creams for a long-time.

- *Stress.* Reducing stress in your life can reduce itching.

- *Scratching.* It is hard to resist scratching, you can try rubbing, pressing or patting the skin. You may need to see a dermatologist (a doctor who specialises in skin conditions) if you are not able to manage the itching yourself.

Anger

Anger is a normal reaction to having a chronic condition. Loss of control over your body and life can make you feel frustrated, helpless and hopeless. You may find yourself asking **'Why me?'** You may be angry with yourself for not taking better care of your health; with your family because they are not supportive enough; or with your doctor because he or she can't 'fix' your problems.

Sometimes your anger may be misplaced when you find yourself shouting at the cat. Misplaced anger is quite common, especially if you are not even aware that you are angry.

To manage your anger, you need to admit that you are angry and find out why or with whom you are angry. You need to find positive ways you can express your anger otherwise the anger can build up and you may upset other people or make your condition worse. Built up anger can not only become explosive and offend others, it can also turn inward and intensify the experience of other symptoms of your disease like depression.

39

Managing Anger

- *Communicate your anger in words.* Try not to blame or upset other people. Learn to use "I" messages rather than "you" messages to talk about your feelings (see Chapter 7). Friends and relatives may not be able to help you. Most of us are not very good at dealing with angry people even if the anger is justified. You may need to seek counselling or join a patient support group.

- *Change your expectations.* You can't expect to get completely better, but you can expect that you will still be able to do many pleasurable things. You will be able to slow down the decline of your illness and may be able to stop it getting worse. Don't think about the 10% of things you can't do, think about the 90% of things you still can do. Develop a positive attitude to life.

- *Channel your anger through new activities.* Find new hobbies and activities such as writing, music or painting. Some people find these extremely therapeutic; if not these you might be able to think up something else that suits your interests. Some people find prayer helpful.

Depression

Depression is another common reaction to a chronic illness. Some people say they are "sad", "down" or "feeling low". It may not always be easy to recognise when you are depressed. Even more difficult is recognising when you might be falling into a deep depression. Just as there are many degrees of pain, there are different degrees of depression. Any one with a long-term condition almost certainly would have had some problems with depression. Depression is felt by everyone at some time or the other. It is how you handle it that makes the difference.

There are certain emotions that can lead to depression:

- *Fears and worries about your future.* These may be about finances, the family or the progress of the disease. Constant worry about these issues can lead to depression. Confront them early on. Deal with any specific problem that is making you anxious. Chapter 12 deals with certain decisions we all have to make at some time in our lives. If the issues are clarified in your own mind and with your family, you will find you are less uncertain about the future.

- *Frustration at not being able to do things.* You may find yourself thinking, "I used to be able to do this myself," or "Why doesn't anyone understand me." Thoughts like these can leave you feeling isolated if you keep holding on to them.

- *Feeling you have lost control of your life.* It may come from having to rely on medication, having to count on others to help you perform activities of daily life, or having to visit outpatients on a regular basis.

These feelings are often experienced in combination, making it difficult to understand the root cause of the depression. Sometimes people try to mask their depression by *unrealistic "cheeriness" and refuse to accept offers of help.* But being depressed is not pleasant and people can **learn** to recognise it, accept it and manage it. The first step is to learn to recognise the signs of depression.

Recognising Depression

Here is a list of common signs of depression that you can learn to recognise.

- You feel a *general feeling of unhappiness* that won't go away.

- You feel a *loss of interest in life, not able to enjoy anything, avoiding people, not wanting to answer the doorbell.* Isolation is an important symptom of depression.

- You have lost interest in *personal care and grooming.*

- You find it *hard to make simple decisions.* Unable to concentrate.

- You feel a *loss of energy.* Feel very tired all the time.

- You feel *restless and twitchy.*

- You have lost your appetite and are *losing weight* or are eating more and have *put on weight.*

- You find it *difficult to sleep* or feel you are *sleeping too much.*

- You have gone *off sex.* (Sometimes this can be due to side effects of medication; talk this over with your doctor.)

- You feel useless. There is *loss of self-confidence, low self-image.*

- You get *suicidal thoughts.* If this happens, get help from close friends, a psychologist or a doctor. These feelings will pass and you will feel better, so get help.

- You frequently have *careless accidents,* such as dropping things or bumping into things.

- You feel *irritable.* Get into frequent arguments over minor matters, things that did not bother you before.

- You feel *worse at a certain time of day,* usually in the morning.

Managing Depression

There are things you can do to help yourself:

1. *Check your medicines.* Some medicines such as tranquillisers and narcotic painkillers are 'downers' and make depression worse. Check with your doctor or pharmacist if you think your depression might be a side effect of your medicine.

2. *Alcohol may make depression worse.* Get advice on how to cut down if you think you are drinking too much alcohol.

3. *Keep on with your daily activities.*

4. *Visit and talk with friends.*

5. *Join a group.* Get involved in a local group or join an adult education class.

6. *Volunteer.* People who help other people are hardly ever depressed.

7. *Make plans and carry them out.* Plant a tree.

8. *Go on holiday.* Even a couple of days away with friends or relatives can help. Look out for day trips and tours organised locally.

9. *Do 20 to 30 minutes of physical activity every day.*

10. *Make a list of rewards for yourself.* Listen to your favourite music, plan a trip to the cinema or plan something you can look forward to.

42

11. *Use positive self-talk.*

12. *Get help* **at once** *if you are thinking about suicide or harming yourself. Call immediately a friend, a religious leader, a care professional, local community centre, support agency like the Samaritans or NHS Direct (0845 4647).*

Sleep Problems

When we are asleep, the body can restore itself. Problems with sleep can lead to fatigue. There are things you can do to help you sleep better.

- Get a comfortable bed that allows you to move easily and supports your body well.

- Find a comfortable sleeping position. Try using small pillows to help.

- Raise the head of your bed on wooden blocks by about four to six inches to make breathing easier.

- Keep your bedroom at a warm temperature.

- Use a vaporiser if the air is dry; warm and moist air makes breathing easier.

- Keep a lamp and telephone beside your bed.

Things to Avoid Before Bedtime

- *Eating.* Digesting food takes energy and means that your body will not have the energy resources to restore itself.

- *Alcohol.* Alcohol leads to a shallow sleep and means that you will wake up several times during the night.

- *Caffeine.* Caffeine is a stimulant and can keep you awake. Caffeine is found in coffee, tea, colas and other soft drinks and chocolate.

- *Food with MSG (monosodium glutamate).* Chinese food and pre-packaged meals often contain MSG which can act as a stimulant.

- *Smoking.* Nicotine in cigarettes is a stimulant. Falling asleep with a lit cigarette is a fire hazard.

- *Diet pills.* These contain stimulants.

- *Sleeping pills.* Sleeping pills become less effective over time and are often addictive. If you stop taking them, it becomes even harder to get to sleep.

- *Diuretics (water pills).* Take these medicines in the morning so you are not woken by the need to pass water.

43

Develop a Routine

- Go to bed at the same time and get up at the same time. If you need to, take a nap in the afternoon. Stay awake after your evening meal until you are ready for bed.

- If you want to get back to a normal pattern of sleep (for example if you are going to bed at 4 a.m. and sleeping until noon) you will need to reset your sleep clock. Try to go to bed one hour later or earlier each day until you get to the pattern you want.

- Regular exercise can help you sleep well.

- Get out in the fresh air for a few minutes every day.

- Get used to doing the same things every night before you go to bed. A 'time-to-get-ready-for-bed' routine such as having a bath and reading a chapter in a book helps your body to wind down and relax.

Other Tips

- If you get into bed and can't fall asleep, get up and go into another room until you are sleepy.

- To take your mind off worries, try a distraction technique such as counting backward from 100 by 3's or naming a country for every letter of the alphabet.

- Don't worry about not getting enough sleep. You will sleep if your body needs sleep.

- For people who are religious, doing prayer helps go to sleep.

If you find you are able to get to sleep very easily but are still tired all the time, it may be because you are not breathing properly at night. You may have a sleep disorder such as 'obstructive sleep apnoea'. This should be investigated.

44

Using Your Mind to Manage Symptoms

What we think and feel can make our body react. You can learn how to use the power of your mind to relax; reduce stress and anxiety; and reduce pain.

Relaxation Techniques

We all have ways to relax; we can walk, watch TV or garden. Relaxation techniques are different because they are ways to use your mind to help your body become relaxed. The aim is to turn off the outside world so your mind and body are at rest.

When you practise these techniques try and stick to the following guidelines:

- *Pick a quiet place and time.* Find a place where you will not be disturbed for at least 15 minutes.

- *Practise twice a day.*

- *Be patient.* It may take you three to four weeks before you notice benefits.

- *Try different techniques.* Find a method that helps you, don't use a method you find unpleasant or which makes you anxious.

Muscle Relaxation

Muscle Relaxation is a way to reduce the tension in muscles. Tense muscles can make pain, shortness of breath and stress worse.

Try each of the following three techniques and choose the one that works best for you. It might help you to concentrate if you tape record the script.

1. Progressive Muscle Relaxation

Edmund Jacobson, a physiologist, discovered that to learn how to relax muscles, you need to know what they feel like when they are tense. The first step therefore is to become familiar with the difference between the feeling of tension and the feeling of relaxation.

A short exercise will allow you to compare these feelings. Please pause for about 10 seconds whenever there is a series of dots (....).

Make yourself as comfortable as possible. Loosen any clothing that feels tight. Uncross your legs and ankle. Allow your body to feel supported by the surface on which you are sitting or lying.

Close your eyes. Take a deep breath, filling your chest and breathing all the way down to the abdomen. Hold..... Breathe out through pursed lips, and, as you breathe out, let as much tension as possible flow out with your breath. Let all your muscles feel heavy and let your whole body just sink into the surface beneath you....Good.

This exercise guides you through the major muscle groups, asking you to first tense and then relax those muscles. If you have a pain in a particular area today, tense those muscles only gently or not at all and focus on relaxing them.

Become aware of the muscles in your feet and calves. Pull your toes back up toward your knees. Notice the tension in your feet and calves. Release and relax. Notice the discomfort leaving as relief and warmth replace it. That's it.

Now tighten the muscles of your thighs and buttocks. Hold and feel the tension. Let go and allow the muscles to relax. The relaxed muscles feel heavy and supported by the surface upon which you are sitting or lying.

Tense the muscles in your abdomen and chest. Notice a tendency to hold your breath as you tense. Relax, and notice that it is natural to want to take a deep breath to relieve the tension in this area. Take a deep breath now; breathing all the way down to the abdomen. As you breathe out, allow all the tension to flow out with your breath.

45

Now, stretching your fingers out straight, tense your fingers and tighten your arm muscles. Relax. Feel the tension flowing out as the circulation returns.

Press your shoulder blades together, tightening the muscles in your shoulders and neck. This is a place where many people carry a lot of tension. Hold....Now, let go. Notice how the muscles feel warmer and more alive.

Tighten all the muscles of your face and head. Notice the tension, especially around your eyes and in your jaw. Now relax, allowing your jaw to become slack and slightly open...That's right. Note the difference.

Now take another deep breath, breathing all the way down to the abdomen. And, as you breath out, allow your body to sink heavily into the surface beneath you, becoming even more deeply relaxed. Good.

Enjoy this comfortable feeling of relaxation....Remember it. With practice, you will become skilled at recognising muscle tension and releasing it....

Prepare to come back to the here and now. Take three deep breaths. And, when you're ready, open your eyes.

Once you have learned this technique, you will not need to tense up your body, you will just have to find the area of tension and let it go.

For people who have pain in the joints, progressive muscle relaxation may not be a good technique. If it causes you pain, try another technique.

2. Body Scan

This relaxation technique does not need you to tense or move your muscles. It is best done lying down. First you have to concentrate on your breathing.

After three or four minutes of concentrating on your breathing, move your attention to your toes. Don't move these, just think about how they feel. Don't worry if you don't feel anything at all. If you find any tension there, let it go as you breathe out.

After a few moments of concentrating on your toes, move your attention to the bottoms of your feet. Again, don't move, just concentrate on any sensations you have. Let go of any tension you may find as you breathe out. Next concentrate on the top of your feet and your ankles. After a few more moments, bring your attention to your lower legs.

Continue this process, shifting your attention every few moments to another part of your body, working slowly upward to your head. If you find tension, let it go as you breathe out. If your mind starts to wander, just bring your attention back to the feelings in your body and your breathing.

This technique can also be used to help you get to sleep because it helps to clear your mind of any worries or distracting thoughts. The key is to give your full attention to scanning your body for tension and releasing it.

3. The Relaxation Response

This technique developed by Dr Herbert Benson aims to help your body relax. If your body has been in a constant state of tension and you want to relieve this tension, you will need to bring to your mind a relaxation response. To achieve this, you will first need to create the right environment.

1. *Find a quiet place* where there are few or no distractions.

2. *Find a position in which you can remain comfortable for 20 minutes.*

3. *Choose a word, object or pleasant feeling to think about.* For example, repeat a word or sound like the word "one", look at an object like a flower, or concentrate on a feeling, such as peace.

4. *Adopt a passive attitude.* Empty all thoughts and distractions from your mind. You may become aware of thoughts, images and feelings, but don't concentrate on them. Just allow them to pass by.

Then carry out the following steps to draw out the relaxation response:

1. *Sit quietly* in a comfortable position.

2. *Close your eyes.*

3. *Relax all your muscles,* starting at your feet and working up to your face. Keep them relaxed.

4. *Breathe in through your nose.* Become aware of your breathing. As you breathe out through your mouth, say the word you chose

silently to yourself. Try to empty all thoughts from your mind; concentrate on your word.

5. *Continue* this for 10 to 20 minutes. You may open your eyes to check the time but do not use an alarm. When you finish, sit quietly for several minutes, at first with your eyes closed. Do not stand up for a few minutes.

6. Don't worry about whether you have achieved a deep level of relaxation. *Keep a passive attitude* and let relaxation occur at its own pace. When you get distracting thoughts, ignore them and go back to repeating the word you chose.

7. *Practise* this once or twice a day, but not during the two hours after a meal. Digestion can get in the way of relaxation.

Guided Imagery

Using guided imagery, you can divert your mind from your symptoms and take yourself to another time and place where you will feel deeply relaxed.

You can use the script in any of the following three ways:

1. Read the script several times so that you know what it says. Then sit or lie down in a quiet place and go through it in your mind. The script should take 15 to 20 minutes to complete.

2. Ask a family member or a friend to read you the script slowly. Ask them to pause for about 10 seconds when there is a series of dots (….).

3. Make a tape recording of the script and play it to yourself.

Guided Imagery Script

A Walk in the Country

Make yourself as comfortable as possible, sitting or lying down. Loosen any tight clothing. Uncross your arms, legs and ankles. Allow your body to feel completely supported by the surface on which you are sitting or lying.

Close your eyes.

Take a deep breath in through your nose, breathing all the way down to the abdomen. Hold....Breathe out slowly through slightly pursed lips, and, as you do, relax your whole body, allowing all your muscles to feel limp and heavy....Good.

Scan your body for any muscle tension, starting with your head and passing all the way down to your toes.

Release any tension in your face, head and neck by letting your jaw become slack and your head feel heavy on your shoulders. Allow your shoulders to drop heavily. Take a deep breath and relax your chest and abdomen. Allow your arms and legs to feel heavy and to sink into the surface beneath you.

Now take a deep breath and become aware of any remaining tension in your body. As you breathe out, allow all the muscles of your body to sink heavily into the surface beneath you, becoming even more deeply relaxed....Good.

Imagine yourself walking along an old country lane....the sun is warm on your back and the birds are singing.

Soon, you have come across an old gate. Open it and go through. You find yourself in a meadow. Flowers growing where they've seeded themselves . . . honeysuckle growing in the hedgerow. . . . soft green grasses. Breathe deeply, smelling the flowers. Listen to the birds and insects. Feel the gentle breeze warm against your skin. . . . All of your senses are alive and responding with pleasure to this peaceful time and place.

When you're ready to move on, you slowly follow a path, eventually coming to a more wooded area. The sun is filtered through the leaves. The air feels mild and a little cooler.

Make yourself as comfortable as possible, sitting or lying down. Loosen any tight clothing. Uncross your arms, legs and ankles. Allow your body to feel completely supported by the surface on which you are sitting or lying.

You become aware of the sound and smell of a nearby stream. You pause, breathing deeply of the cool and fragrant air several times, and with each breath you feel more refreshed. Soon, you come to the stream. It is clear and clean as it flows and tumbles over some rocks and some fallen logs.

You follow the path along the stream for a way, and after a while, you come out into a sunlit clearing, where you discover a small waterfall emptying into a quiet pool of water. There is a rainbow in the mist.

You find a comfortable place to sit for a while. A perfect place where you can feel completely relaxed. You feel good as you allow yourself to just enjoy the warmth and solitude of this peaceful place.

After a while, you become aware that it's time to return. You walk back down the path through the cool and fragrant trees, out into the sun-drenched meadow, one last smell of the flowers and out the gate.

You leave this secret retreat for now and return down the lane, noticing you feel calm and rested. You know that you can visit this special place whenever you wish to take some time to refresh yourself and renew your energy.

When you are ready to, take three deep breaths and open your eyes.

Visualisation

This technique is similar to guided imagery. It is another way to use your mind to imagine yourself any way you want, doing things you want to do.
Some examples are:

- Remember pleasant scenes from your past. Try to remember every detail of a special holiday or party that made you happy.

- Plan how you would spend a million pounds. What would your ideal home or garden look like?

- Use your mind to think of symbols for the pain felt in a part of your body. For example a painful joint might be red or a tight chest might have a tight band round it. Then try to change these images. The red colour might fade away, or the tight band might stretch and stretch until it falls off.

- Use visualisation when you are writing your action plan. Imagine yourself doing your exercises or eating a healthy diet.

People have found that they can reduce the pain and distress of symptoms by changing unpleasant images to pleasant ones.

Distraction

This is a way of training your mind to move attention away from your symptoms. It does not mean that you ignore the symptoms, but that you choose not to think about them. Using your mind works best for short activities or for times when you know your symptoms will be a problem. Try one of the following distraction techniques:

1. Make plans for what you will do after the unpleasant activity. For example, if climbing stairs is painful, think about what you will do when you get to the top.

2. Think of a person's name, a flower or whatever you like for every letter of the alphabet. If you get stuck on one letter go on to the next.

3. Count backwards from 100 by threes (100, 97, 94…)

4. To help yourself get through housework (such as sweeping, mopping or vacuuming), imagine your floor is a map of the world. Try naming all the countries moving east to west or north to south. If

you are not very good at geography, imagine your favourite shopping centre and where each shop is to be found.

5. Try to remember the words to your favourite songs or all the characters in your favourite TV soap opera or in a favourite film.

You can also use distraction for symptoms which last for a long time, like depression or chronic pain. You can do this by using your mind for carrying out an activity that interests you such as cooking, reading or going to the cinema.

Self-Talk and Positive Thinking

We all talk to ourselves all the time. We think things like, "I'm so tired, I don't want to cook tonight." Or "I'm so glad I saw this film last night, it was such fun." These thoughts are called 'self-talk'. Some self-talk is negative, about our doubts and fears and about whether we will be able to cope with our condition. Negative thoughts can make symptoms like pain, depression and tiredness feel much worse. You can learn to make self-talk work for you and change unhelpful thoughts to helpful ones which will help you manage your symptoms better.

Changing the way you think needs practise.

1. Listen carefully to what you say to yourself or about yourself. Write down all the negative self-talk statements. Pay attention to the things you say during times that are very difficult for you. For example, what do you say to yourself when you get up in the morning with pain or at the times you are feeling low?

2. Work on changing each negative statement to a positive one. For example:

Negative statement	Positive statement
I don't want to get up; I'm too tired	I have the energy to get up and do the things I enjoy
I can't do the things I like anymore, so why bother	I know I can do anything I believe I can
I'm good for nothing	Other people need and depend on me; I'm worthwhile

3. Read and speak out loud these statements. Repeating them will help you replace the old negative statements.

4. Practise the new statements in real situations. With time, they will become your natural way of thinking.

Mindful Meditation

There are many types of meditation. Meditation is a part of most religious or spiritual tradition. It is a way to quiet the mind and can also help you to quiet the body and manage pain, stress, tiredness or shortness of breath. Mindful meditation is one type of meditation. It is quite simple. To do mindful meditation, you need a quiet place and about five minutes. You can sit in a chair with your feet flat on the ground and your hands in your lap or on your knees. If you wish and are able to, you can sit on the floor with legs crossed or in a more traditional yoga position. You must sit in the way most comfortable to you.

The essence of mindful meditation is to concentrate on your breathing. It is best if you can do diaphragmatic or belly breathing, but you do not have to take deep breaths.

You will need to breathe taking the following steps:

1. Keep your full attention on your breathing.

2. Breathe in slowly; hold your breath for a moment; then breathe out slowly.

3. If your mind wanders or you become very aware of a part of your body such as an itch, bring your thoughts back to your breathing. If you become uncomfortable in your sitting position, still concentrate on the breathing. In many cases you will find that the discomfort goes away. If it continues, scratch the itch or change your sitting position. As you do this, pay full attention to what you are doing. In mindful meditation, it is important to be fully aware of what you are doing at a specific moment!

At first, you may only be able to do this for a few minutes, but with practise, you will improve. If you practise mindful meditation for 15 to 30 minutes a day, four or five times a week, you will find that over time this can be a great symptom management tool.

Prayer

Many people with chronic illness find prayer helpful. It is helpful in managing both the physical and emotional symptoms of their disease. For some, it helps to reduce tension and anxiety and for others it helps to take their thoughts away from their symptoms. Prayer is the oldest of all symptom management techniques.

Remember the Key Principles of Symptom Management

- *Symptoms have many causes.* This means there are many ways to manage most symptoms. You need to learn what causes your symptoms.

- *Not all ways of managing symptoms will work for everyone.* Find out what works best for you. Be flexible. Keep checking on which technique works best for which symptoms and under what circumstances.

- *Give yourself several weeks* to practise new skills.

- Be patient and *try not to give up.*

- If using any of the techniques upsets you, then stop using it and try another.

54

Tips for Using Symptom-Management Techniques

- **Choose a technique to try first.** Give this method a fair trial. Practise it twice a day for at least two weeks before deciding whether it works for you or not.

- **Try some other techniques, giving each the same trial period.** It is important to try several techniques. Only after trying a few you will be able to determine your own preferences.

- **Think about when you will use each technique you have chosen.** For example, some of the methods may require substantial lifestyle changes. Eventually it is best to use a combination of techniques depending on different needs that may arise at different times: horses for courses.

- **Practice is important for mastering any skill.** Place stickers or notes to remind you to practise regularly and master the skills.

- **Try linking the practise of each technique with some other established activity in your daily routine.** For example, practise relaxation immediately after brushing your teeth. Also you could ask a friend or family member to remind you to practise; they might even want to participate.

• • •

Suggested Further Reading

Ball, Nigel, and Nich Hough. *The Sleep Solution: A 21-Night Program for Restful Sleep.* Berkeley, Calif.: Ulysses Press, 1998.

Bernard, Jeffrey D. *Itch Mechanisms and Management of Pruritus.* New York: McGraw-Hill, 1994.

Burns, David D. *The Feeling Good Handbook.* New York: NAL/Dutton, 1999.

Carter, Les, and Frank Minirth. *The Anger Workbook: A 13-Step Interactive Plan.* Nashville, Tenn.: Thomas Nelson, 1993.

Catalano, Ellen M., and Kimeron N. Hardin. *The Chronic Pain Control Work Book: A Step-By-Step Guide to Coping With and Overcoming Pain.* Berkeley, Calif.: New Harbinger, 1996.

Chalder, Trudie. *Coping with Chronic Fatigue.* London: Sheldon Press.

Cousins, Norman. *Head First: The Biology of Hope and the Healing Power of the Human Spirit.* New York: E. P. Dutton, 1989.

Craze, Richard. *Teach Yourself Relaxation.* Chicago: Contemporary Publishing, 1998.

Cunningham, J. Barton, and Bart Cunningham. *The Stress Management Sourcebook: Everything You Need To Know.* Chicago: Contemporary Publishing, 1997.

Davis, Martha. *The Relaxation Production Workshop, 5th Ed.* Berkeley, Cal.: New Harbinger, 2000.

Dossey, Larry. *Prayer Is Good Medicine.* San Francisco: HarperCollins, 1996.

Gilbert, Paul. *Overcoming Depression.* Revised Ed. Constable Robinson, 2000.

Hanley, J.L. and Nancy Deville. *Tired of Being Tired.* London: Michael Joseph, 2002.

Hauck, Paul. *Calm Down.* London: Sheldon Press, 1980.

Johnston, Fiona. *Getting a Good Night's Sleep.* London: Sheldon Press, 2000.

Kabat-Zinn, Jon. *Wherever You Go, There You Are: Mindfulness Meditation in Everyday Life.* New York: Hyperion, 1995.

55

Lewinsohn, Peter, with Ricardo Munoz, Mary Youngren, and Antoinette Zeiss. *Control Your Depression.* New York: Simon and Schuster, 1992.

McKay, Matthew, and Patrick Fanning. *The Daily Relaxer.* Oakland, Calif.: New Harbinger, 1997.

Natelson, Benjamin H. *Facing and Fighting Fatigue: A Practical Approach.* New Haven, Conn.: Yale University Press, 1998.

Ornstein, Robert, and David Sobel. *Healthy Pleasures.* Reading, Mass.: Addison-Wesley, 1990.

Peale, Norman V. *Positive Imaging: The Powerful Way to Change Your Life.* New York: Ballantine Books, 1996.

Pascualy, Ralph, et al. *Snoring and Sleep Apnea.* Demos Medical Publications, 2000.

Shealy, C. Norman. *90 Days to Stress Free Living.* Element Books Inc., 1999.

Sheller, Mary Dale. *Growing Older, Feeling Better in Body, Mind and Spirit.* Palo Alto, Calif.: Bull Publishing Co., 1993.

Shone, Neville. *Coping Successfully with Pain.* London: Sheldon Press, 2000.

Tannen, Deborah. *You Just Don't Understand: Men and Women in Conversation.* London: Virago, 1992.

Williams, Christopher J. *Overcoming Depression.* Sevenoaks, England: Arnold, 2001.

Zammit, Gary. *Good Nights: How to Stop Sleep Deprivation, Overcome Insomnia and Get the Sleep You Need.* Kansas City, Mo.: Andrew McMeel Publishing, 1997.

CHAPTER
4

Exercising for Fun and Fitness

"The weakest and oldest among us can become some sort of athlete, but only the strongest can survive as spectators. Only the hardiest can withstand the perils of inertia, inactivity, and immobility."

J H Bland and S M Cooper,
Semin Arthritis Rheum:1984

REGULAR EXERCISE AND PHYSICAL ACTIVITY ARE VITAL to your physical and emotional health and can bring you fun and fitness at the same time. Having a chronic illness and growing older can make an active lifestyle seem far away. Some people have never been very active and others have given up leisure activities because of illness.

Unfortunately, long periods of inactivity in anyone can lead to weakness, stiffness, fatigue, poor appetite, high blood pressure, obesity, osteoporosis, constipation, and increased sensitivity to pain, anxiety, and depression. These problems arise from chronic illnesses as well. So, it can be difficult to tell whether it is the illness, inactivity, or a combination of the two that is responsible for these problems. Although we do not have cures for many of these illnesses yet, we do know the cure for inactivity—exercise!

Most people have a sense that exercising and being active is healthier and more satisfying than being inactive, but often have a hard time finding information and support to get started on a more active way of life.

Thanks to the knowledge gained from many people with chronic illnesses who have worked with health professionals in exercise research, we can now advise on exercise for fun and fitness, as well as exercise for helping manage your illnesses and for making everyday activities less stressful.

In this chapter, you will learn how to improve your health and fitness and make wise exercise choices. However, this advice is not intended to take the place of therapeutic recommendations from health professionals. If you've had an exercise plan prescribed for you that differs from the suggestions here, take this book to your doctor or physiotherapist and ask what she or he thinks about this programme. Later in this book, we will provide additional information and helpful exercise ideas for people with specific chronic illnesses.

Regular exercise benefits everyone, especially people with chronic health problems. Regular exercise improves levels of strength, energy, and self-confidence, and lessens anxiety and depression. Exercise can help maintain a good weight, which takes stress off weight-bearing joints and improves blood pressure, blood sugar, and blood fat levels. There is evidence that regular exercise can help to "thin" the blood, or prevent blood clots, which is one of the reasons exercise can be of particular benefit to people with heart disease, cerebrovascular disease, and peripheral vascular disease.

In addition, strong muscles can help people with arthritis to protect their joints by improving stability and absorbing shock. Regular exercise also helps nourish joints and keep cartilage and bone healthy. Regular exercise has been shown to help people with chronic lung disease improve endurance and reduce shortness of breath (and the number of trips to Accident and Emergency [A & E] services). Many people with claudication (leg pain from severe atherosclerotic constriction in the arteries of the lower extremities) can walk farther without leg pain after undertaking a regular exercise programme. Studies of people with heart disease who exercise in cardiac rehabilitation programmes suggest that exercise may even increase life expectancy. Regular exercise is an important part of controlling blood sugar levels, losing weight, and reducing the risks of cardiovascular complications for people with diabetes.

The good news is that it doesn't take hours of painful, sweat-soaked exercise to achieve most of these health benefits. Even short periods of gentle physical activity can significantly improve health and fitness, reduce disease risks, and give your mood a boost.

Exercise reconditions your body, helping to restore function previously lost owing to inactivity and illness. This will help you improve your health, feel better, and manage your chronic illness better. Feeling more in control and less at the mercy of your chronic illness is one of the biggest and best benefits of becoming an exercise self-manager.

Developing an Active Lifestyle

Right, so you want to be more physically active. One way is to set aside a special time for a formal exercise programme, involving such planned activities as walking, jogging, swimming, tennis, aerobic dance, exercise to an exercise videotape, and so on. But don't underestimate the value and importance of just being more physically active throughout the day as you carry out your usual activities. Both can be helpful.

The formal programmes are usually more visible and get more attention. But being more physical in everyday life can also pay off. Consider taking the stairs a floor or two instead of waiting impatiently for a lift. When travelling to work or going shopping by car, park several hundred yards away and walk the remaining distance, rather than trying to find a nearby parking space. Mow the lawn, work in the garden, or just get up once in a while and walk around the house.

These types of daily activities, often not viewed as "exercise," can add up to significant health benefits. Recent studies show that even small amounts of daily activity can raise fitness levels, decrease heart disease risk, and positively alter mood . . . and the activities can be pleasurable, enjoyable ones! Playing with the children, dancing, gardening, bowls, golf . . . all these enjoyable activities can make a big difference. One person commented that she *never* exercised. When asked why she went line dancing several times a week she replied, "Oh, that's not exercise, that's fun." The average day is filled with excellent opportunities to be more physical.

Developing an Exercise Programme

For many people, however, a more formal exercise programme can be helpful. This usually involves setting aside a period of time, at least several times a week, to deliberately focus on increasing fitness. A complete, balanced exercise programme should help you improve these three aspects of fitness:

1. *Flexibility.* This refers to the ability of the joints and muscles to move comfortably through a full, normal range of motion. Limited flexibility can cause pain, increase risk of injury, and make muscles less efficient. Flexibility tends to diminish with inactivity, age, and certain diseases, but you can increase or maximise your flexibility by doing gentle stretching exercises like those described later in Chapter 5.

2. *Strength.* Muscles need to be exercised to maintain their strength. With inactivity, muscles tend to weaken and shrink (atrophy). The weaker the muscles get, the less we feel like using them, and the more inactive we tend to become, creating a vicious circle. Much of the disability and lack of mobility for

people with chronic illness is due to muscle weakness. This weakness can be reversed with a programme of gradually increasing exercise.

3. *Endurance.* Our ability to sustain activity depends on certain vital capacities. The heart and lungs must work efficiently to distribute oxygen-rich blood to the muscles. The muscles must be conditioned to use the oxygen.

Aerobic (meaning "with oxygen") exercise improves this cardiovascular and muscular conditioning. This type of exercise uses the large muscles of your body in a rhythmical, continuous activity. The most effective activities involve your whole body: walking, swimming, dancing, mowing the lawn, and so on. Aerobic exercise improves cardiovascular fitness, lessens heart attack risk, and helps control weight. Aerobic exercise also promotes a sense of well-being . . . easing depression and anxiety, promoting restful sleep, and improving mood and energy levels.

Your Fitness Programme

A complete fitness programme combines exercises to improve each of the three aspects of fitness: flexibility, strength, and endurance. Chapter 5 explains and illustrates a number of flexibility and strengthening exercises. Chapter 6 contains information about endurance or aerobic exercise. If you haven't exercised regularly in some time, or have pain, stiffness, shortness of breath, or weakness that interferes with your daily activities, it is a good idea to discuss your ideas about increasing your exercise with health professionals. Begin your fitness programme by choosing a number of flexibility and strengthening exercises that you are willing to do every day or every other day. Once you are able to comfortably exercise for at least 10 minutes at a time, you are ready to start adding some endurance or aerobic activities.

Many people wonder how to choose the right exercises and how to know what's best for them. The truth is that the best exercises for you are the ones that will help you do what you want to do. Often, the most important decision to start a successful fitness programme is to choose a goal (something you want to do) that exercise can help you reach. Once you have a goal in mind, it is much easier to choose exercises that make sense to you. There is no doubt that we all are more successful exercisers if we know where we want exercise to take us. If you don't see how exercise can be helpful to you, it is hard to get excited about adding just another task to our days.

Choose Your Goal and Make a Plan

1. **Choose a goal** that you want to do but don't or can't do now because of some physical reason. For example, you might want to enjoy a shopping or fishing expedition with your friends, mow the lawn, or take a family holiday.

2. **Think about why you can't or don't do it or enjoy doing it now.** It might be that you get tired before everybody else, that it's too hard to get up from a low chair or bench, that climbing steps is painful or makes your legs tired, or that your shoulders are too weak or stiff to cast your fishing line or carry a heavy bag.

3. **Decide what about your abilities makes it difficult to do what you want.** For example, if getting up from a low seat is difficult, you may realise that your hips, knees, or joints are stiff and that your leg muscles are weak. In this case, look for flexibility and strengthening exercises for hips and knees. If you decide a major problem is that your shoulders are stiff and your arms too weak to handle a heavy bag, choose flexibility and strengthening exercises for your shoulders and arms.

4. **Design your exercise plan.** Choose no more than 10–12 exercises at first. Start by doing 3–5 repetitions of each and review the information in Chapter 5. As you get comfortable, you can increase repetitions and kinds of exercise. If you want to improve your endurance, read over Chapter 6 about aerobic exercise. Start off with short periods and build up gradually. Health and fitness take time to build, but every day you exercise you are healthier and on your way to fitness. That's why it's so important to make sure you keep it up.

What Are Your Exercise Barriers?

Health and fitness make sense. Yet, when faced with actually being more physically active, most people can come up with scores of excuses, concerns, and worries. These barriers can prevent us from even taking the first step. Here are some common barriers and possible solutions:

"I don't have enough time." Everyone has the same amount of time. We just choose to use it differently. It's a matter of priorities. Some find a lot of time for television, but nothing to spare for fitness. It doesn't really take a lot of time.

Even five minutes a day is a good start, and it's much better than no physical activity. You may be able to combine activities, like watching television while pedalling a stationary bicycle, or arranging "walking meetings" to discuss business or family matters.

"I'm too tired." When you're out of shape, you feel listless and tend to tire easily. Then you don't exercise because you're tired, and this becomes yet another vicious cycle. You have to break out of the "too tired" cycle. Regular physical activity increases your stamina and gives you more energy to do the things you like. As you get back into shape, you will recognise the difference between feeling listless or "out of shape" and feeling physically tired.

"I'm too old." You're never too old for some type of physical activity. No matter what your level of fitness is or your age, you can always find some ways to increase activity, energy, and sense of well-being. To date our oldest self-manager has been 99. Fitness is especially important as we age.

"I'm too ill." It may be true that you are too ill for a vigorous or strenuous exercise programme, but you can usually find some ways to be more active. Remember, you can exercise one minute at a time, several times a day. The enhanced physical fitness can help you better cope with your illness and prevent further problems.

"I get enough exercise." This may be true, but for most people, their jobs and daily activities do not provide enough sustained exercise to keep them fully fit and energetic.

"Exercise is boring." You can make it more interesting and fun. Exercise with other people. Entertain yourself with a headset and audio tapes or listen to the radio. Vary your activities and your walking routes.

"Exercise is painful." The old saying "No pain, no gain" is simply wrong and out-of-date. Recent evidence shows that significant health benefits come from gentle, low-intensity, enjoyable physical activity. You may sweat, or feel a bit short of breath, but if you feel more pain when you finish than before you started, take a close look at what you are doing. More likely than not, you are either exercising improperly or overdoing it for your particular condition. Talk to your instructor, physiotherapist, or doctor. You may simply need to be less vigorous or change the type of exercise that you're doing.

"I'm too embarrassed." For some, the thought of putting on a skintight, "designer" exercise outfit and prancing around in public is delightful, but for others it is downright distressing. Fortunately, as we'll describe, the options for physical activity range from exercise in the privacy of your own home to group social activities. You should be able to find something that suits you.

"I'm afraid I'll have a heart attack." In most cases, the risk of a heart attack may be greater for those who are not physically active than for those who exercise

regularly. But if you are worried about this, consult your doctor. Especially if your illness is under control, it's probably safer to exercise than *not* to exercise.

"It's too cold, it's too hot, it's too dark, etc." If you are flexible, and vary your type of exercise, you can generally work around the changes in weather that make certain types of exercise more difficult. Consider indoor activities like using an exercise bicycle or walking through a museum or shopping mall.

"I'm afraid I won't be able to do it right or be successful. I'm afraid I'll fail." Many people don't start a new project because they are afraid they will fail or not be able to finish it successfully. If you feel this way about starting an exercise programme, remember two things. Firstly, whatever activities you are able to do—no matter how short or "easy"—will be much better for you than doing nothing. Be proud of what you *have* done, not guilty about what you *haven't* done. Secondly, new projects often seem overwhelming—until we get started and learn to enjoy each day's adventures and successes.

Perhaps you have come up with some other barriers. The human mind is incredibly creative. But you can turn that creativity to your advantage by using it to come up with even better ways to refute the excuses and develop positive attitudes about exercise and fitness. If you get stuck, ask others for suggestions, or try some of the self-talk suggestions in Chapter 3.

Preparing to Exercise

Working out how to make the commitment of time and energy to regular exercise is a challenge for everyone. If you have a chronic illness, you have even more challenges. You must take precautions and find a safe and comfortable programme. Even with a chronic illness, most people can do some kind of aerobic exercise.

If your illness is not fairly stable, if you have been inactive for more than six months, if you have a heart condition, or if you have questions about starting an aerobic exercise programme, it is best to consult your doctor or physiotherapist first. Take this book with you when you discuss your exercise ideas, or prepare a list of your specific questions.

People with arthritis, for example, should understand how to adapt their exercise to changes in their arthritis and joint problems. People with heart disease or respiratory disease should not "exercise through" potentially serious symptoms, such as chest pain, palpitations (irregular heartbeats), shortness of breath, or excessive fatigue. They should notify their doctors of any significant worsening of their usual symptoms or if new symptoms appear. Resumption of exercise should begin only after getting the doctor's clearance to do so. Also, don't exercise when you are experiencing flu symptoms, an upset stomach, diarrhoea, or other acute illnesses.

63

Learning how much to push yourself while exercising, without doing "too much," is especially important.

We hope that this chapter will help you gain knowledge to meet these challenges and enjoy the benefits of physical fitness. Start by learning your individual needs and limits. If possible, talk to your doctor and other health professionals who understand your kind of chronic illness. Listen to their ideas about special exercise needs and precautions. Learn to be aware of your body, and plan activities accordingly.

Respect your body. If you feel acutely ill, don't exercise. If you can't comfortably complete your warm-up period of flexibility and strengthening exercises, then don't try to do more vigorous conditioning exercises. Your personal exercise programme should be based on *your* current level of health and fitness, *your* goals and desires, *your* abilities and special needs, and *your* likes and dislikes. Deciding to improve your fitness, and feeling the satisfaction of success, has nothing to do with competition or comparing yourself to others.

Opportunities in Your Community

Most people who exercise regularly do so with at least one other person. Two or more people can keep each other motivated, and a whole class can build a feeling of camaraderie. On the other hand, exercising alone gives you the most freedom. You may feel that there are no classes that would work for you or no friend with whom to exercise. If so, start your own programme; as you progress, you may find that these feelings change.

A number of disease-specific voluntary organisations recommend exercise programmes. You can use their helpline numbers to find out about these. In some cases there are local branches meeting in local venues.

There is a wealth of tai chi, yoga, and other courses available in most communities. They are most often offered by your local Further Education College, but there are also many private tutors.

Most local authorities have leisure and recreation departments that run leisure centres. These include swimming pools, exercise suites, badminton, squash, and other indoor sports courts. They are also where many specialist groups meet. These are well worth exploring. There are always qualified instructors about who will talk to you about your personal needs even if you are starting from a very basic point. Their professional qualifications include studies of the needs of people with chronic conditions. By and large, classes and gyms are not expensive. In a few places, doctors can prescribe leisure centre courses.

Hospitals commonly offer medically supervised exercise classes for people with heart or lung disease (cardiac and pulmonary rehabilitation classes). Occasionally, people with other chronic illnesses can be included as well. These programmes are always free and have the advantage of medical supervision, if that's important to you.

Health and fitness clubs usually offer aerobic studios, weight training, cardio-vascular equipment, and sometimes a heated pool. For all these services the fees can be high. The more luxurious the centre, the higher the price. Sometimes these facilities are available at quite reasonable prices to local people at four-star and five-star hotels. The key thing for a beginner to ask about is low-impact programmes (for over 50s if this is appropriate). The qualifications of the staff can vary, so the key is to find an atmosphere and staff who you find sympathetic. As a rule, gyms that emphasise weight lifting generally don't have programmes or personnel to help you with flexible, overall fitness programmes. These are some of the qualities to look for:

1. Classes designed for *moderate and low-intensity* exercise and for beginners. You should be able to observe classes and participate in at least one class before signing up and paying.
2. Instructors with *qualifications and experience.* Knowledgeable instructors are more likely to understand special needs and be willing and able to work with you.
3. Membership policies and fees that suit your diary and financial circumstances.
4. Facilities that are *easy to get to, park near, and enter.* Dressing rooms and exercise sites should be accessible and safe, with professional staff on site.
5. A pool timetable that allows you to follow your programme. For example, some pools have times that are reserved for swimmers (rather than families). Some have women-only sessions.
6. Staff and other members whom you *feel comfortable* being around.

One last note: There are many excellent videotapes for use at home. These vary in intensity, from very gentle chair exercises to more strenuous aerobic exercise. Ask your doctor, physiotherapist, or disease-specific voluntary organisation for suggestions, or review the tapes yourself.

Putting Your Programme Together

The best way to enjoy and keep up your exercise programme is to *suit yourself!* Choose what you want to do, a place where you feel comfortable, and an exercise time that fits your schedule. A woman who wants to have dinner on the table at 6 won't keep up an exercise programme that requires her to leave home for a 5 o'clock class. A retired man who enjoys lunch with friends and an afternoon nap is wise to choose an early- or mid-morning exercise time.

Pick two or three activities you think you would enjoy and that wouldn't put undue stress on your body. Choose activities that can be easily worked into your daily routine. If an activity is new to you, try it out before going to the expense of buying equipment or joining a health club. By having more than one exercise, you can keep active while adapting to holidays, seasons, and changing problems with your condition. Variety also helps keep you from getting bored.

Having fun and enjoying yourself are benefits of exercise that often go unmentioned. Too often we think of exercise as serious business. However, most people who stay with a programme do so because they enjoy it. *They think of their exercise as recreation rather than a chore.* Start off with success in mind. Allow yourself time to get used to new experiences and meet new people. You'll probably find that you look forward to exercise.

Some well-meaning health professionals can make it hard for a person with a chronic illness to stick to an exercise programme. You may have been told simply to "exercise more on your own." The "how" and "when" of that exercise plan, in fact, may have been left entirely up to you. No wonder so many people never start or give up so quickly! Not many of us would make a commitment to do something we don't fully understand. Experience, practice, and success help us establish a habit. Follow the self-management steps in Chapter 1 to make beginning your programme easier.

1. *Keep your exercise goal in mind.* Review "Choose Your Goal and Make a Plan" earlier in this chapter (page 61).
2. *Choose exercises you want to do.* Combine activities that move you toward your goal and those recommended by your health professionals. Select exercises and activities from the next two chapters to get started.
3. *Choose the time and place to exercise.* Tell your family and friends about your plan.
4. *Make an action plan with yourself.* Decide how long you'll continue with these particular exercises. Six to eight weeks is a reasonable time commitment for a new programme.
5. *Make an exercise diary or calendar,* whichever suits you. A

diary or journal will let you record more information. Some people enjoy having a record of what they did and how they felt. For others, a simple calendar on which to note an exercise session is plenty of paperwork. Choose what you like; the point is to have fun and enjoy being active.

6. *Do some self-tests to keep track of your progress.* You will find these at the end of the next two chapters. Record the date and results of the ones you choose.

7. *Start your programme.* Remember to begin gradually and proceed slowly, especially if you haven't exercised in a while.

8. *Repeat the self-tests* at regular intervals, record the results, and check the changes.

9. *Revise your programme.* At the end of your 6–8 weeks, decide what you liked, what worked, and what made exercising difficult. Modify your programme and contract for another few weeks. You may decide to change some exercises, the place or time you exercise, or your exercise partner(s).

10. *Reward yourself for a job well done.* Many people who start an exercise programme find that the rewards come with improved fitness and endurance. Being able to enjoy family outings, a refreshing walk, or trips to the shops, the library, a concert, or a museum are great rewards to look forward to.

67

Keeping It Up

If you haven't exercised recently, you'll undoubtedly experience some new feelings and discomfort in the early days. It's normal to feel muscle tension and possible tenderness around joints, and to be a little more tired in the evenings. *Muscle or joint pain that lasts more than two hours after the exercise, or feeling tired into the next day, means that you have probably done too much too soon. Don't stop;* just exercise less vigorously or for a shorter amount of time the next day.

When you do aerobic exercise, it's natural to feel your heart beat faster, your breathing speed up, and your body get warmer. However, feeling chest pain, excessive shortness of breath, nausea, or dizziness is not what you want. If this happens to you, stop exercising and discontinue your programme until you check with your doctor. (See Table 4.1.)

People who have a chronic illness often have *additional sensations* to sort out. It can be difficult at first to work out whether it is the illness or the exercise or

Table 4.1 *Advice for Exercise Problems*

Problem	Advice
Irregular or very rapid heartbeats	Stop exercising. Check your pulse. Are the beats regular or irregular? How fast is your heartbeat? Make a note of these and discuss this information with your doctor before exercising again. (See page 94)
Pain, tightness, or pressure in the chest, jaw, arms, neck, or back	Stop exercising. Talk to your doctor. Don't exercise until it has been cleared by your doctor.
Unusual, extreme shortness of breath, persisting 10 minutes after you exercise	Notify your doctor and get clearance before exercising again.
Light-headedness, dizziness, fainting, cold sweat, or confusion	Lie down with your feet up, or sit down and put your head between your legs. Check with your doctor before you exercise again.
Excessive tiredness after exercise, especially if you're still tired 24 hours after you exercise	Don't exercise so vigorously next time. If the excessive tiredness persists, check with your doctor. Talk to your doctor before you exercise again.

both that is causing them. Talking to someone else with the illness who has had experience starting a new exercise programme can be a big help. Once you've sorted out the new sensations, you'll be able to exercise with confidence.

Expect setbacks. During the first year, people average two to three interruptions in their exercise schedule, often because of minor injuries or illnesses unrelated to their exercise. You may find yourself sidelined or derailed temporarily. Don't be discouraged. Try a different activity or simply rest. When you are feeling better, resume your programme, but begin at a lower, more gentle level. As a rule of thumb, it will take you the same amount of time to get back into shape as you were out. For instance, if you missed three weeks, it may take at least that long to get back to your previous level. Go slowly. Be kind to yourself. You're in this for the long haul.

Think of your head as the coach and your body as your team. For success, all parts of the team need attention. Be a good coach. *Encourage and praise yourself.* Design activities you feel your team can execute successfully. Choose places that are safe and hospitable. A good coach knows his or her team, sets good goals, and helps the team succeed. A good coach is loyal. A good coach does not belittle, nag, or make anyone feel guilty. Be a good coach to your team.

69

Besides a good coach, everyone needs an enthusiastic cheerleader or two. Of course, you can be your own cheerleader, but being both coach and cheerleader is a lot to do. Successful exercisers usually have at least one *family member* or close friend who actively *supports* their exercise habit. Your cheerleader can exercise with you, help you get other chores done, praise your accomplishments, or just consider your exercise time when making plans. Sometimes cheerleaders pop up by themselves, but don't be bashful about asking for a hand.

With exercise experience you develop a sense of control over yourself and your chronic illness. You learn how to *vary your activities to fit in with your day-to-day needs.* You know when to do less and when to do more. You know that a change in symptoms or a period of inactivity is usually only temporary and doesn't have to be devastating. You know you have the tools to get back on track again.

Give your exercise plan a chance to succeed. Set reasonable goals and enjoy your success. Stay motivated. When it comes to your personal fitness programme, sticking to it and doing it your way makes you a clear winner.

• • •

Suggested Further Reading

Dagleish, Julia. *Health and Fitness Handbook*. London: Longman, 2001.

Hawkins, Jerald. *Walking for Fun and Fitness*. Belmont, Cal.: Wadsworth, 2000.

Rizzo, Terrie. *Fresh Start: The Stanford Medical School Health and Fitness Program*. San Francisco: KQED Books, 1996. Order from: Stanford University HIP, 1000 Welch Road, Palo Alto, CA 94394. Call 650-723-9649 for information.

White, Martha. *Water Exercise: 78 Safe and Effective Exercises for Fitness and Therapy*. Champaign, Ill.: Human Kinetics, 1995.

CHAPTER 5

Exercising for Flexibility and Strength: Warm-Up/Cool-Down

YOU CAN USE THE EXERCISES IN THIS CHAPTER IN SEVERAL WAYS: to get in shape for more vigorous aerobic exercise, on days when you don't do aerobic exercise, and as part of your warm-up and cool-down routines. Choose exercises to build a strengthening and flexibility programme for the whole body.

The exercises are arranged in order from the head and neck down to the toes. Most of the upper-body exercises may be done either sitting or standing. Exercises done lying down can be performed on the floor or on a firm mattress. We have labeled the exercises that are particularly important for good posture "VIP" *(Very Important for Posture)*.

You might enjoy creating a routine of exercises that flow together. Arrange them so that you don't have to get up and down too often. Exercising to gentle, rhythmical music can also add to your enjoyment.

These helpful tips apply to all the exercises that follow:

- *Move slowly and gently.* Do not bounce or jerk.
- To loosen tight muscles and limber up stiff joints, stretch *just until you feel tension,* hold for 5 to 10 seconds, and then relax.
- *Don't push your body until it hurts.* Stretching should feel good, not painful.
- *Start with no more than 5 repetitions* of any exercise. Take at least *2 weeks* to increase to 10 repetitions.
- Always do the *same number* of exercises for your left side as for your right.

- *Breathe naturally.* Do not hold your breath. Count out loud to make sure you are breathing easily.
- If you feel increased symptoms that last more than *2 hours* after exercising, next time do fewer repetitions, or eliminate an exercise that seems to be causing the symptoms. *Don't abandon exercising.*
- *All exercises can be adapted for individual needs.* The following exercises are designed and pictured to include both sides of the body and full range of motion. If you are limited by muscle weakness or joint tightness, go ahead and do the exercise as completely as you can. ***The benefit of doing an exercise comes from moving toward a certain position, not from being able to complete the movement perfectly.*** In some cases you may find that after a while you can complete the movement. At other times, you will continue to perform your own version.

Neck Exercises

1. Heads Up *(VIP)*

This exercise relieves jaw, neck, and upper back tension or pain, and is the start of good posture. You can do it while sitting at a desk, sewing, reading, or exercising. Just sit or stand straight and gently slide your chin back. Keep looking forward as your chin moves backward. You'll feel the back of your neck lengthen and straighten. To help, put your finger on your nose and then draw straight back from your finger. (Don't worry about a little double chin—you really look much better with your neck straight!)

Clues for finding the correct position:

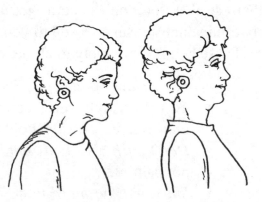

1. Ear over shoulder, *not* out in front
2. Head balanced over neck and trunk, *not* in the lead
3. Back of neck more vertical, not leaning forward
4. Bit of double chin

2. Neck Stretch

In heads-up position (Exercise 1) and with your shoulders relaxed:

   a. Turn slowly to look over your right shoulder. Then turn slowly to look over your left shoulder.

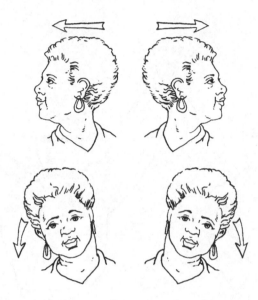

   b. Tilt your head to the right and then to the left. Move your ear toward your shoulder. Do *not* move your shoulder up to your ear.

Don't do these exercises if they cause neck pain, or pain or numbness in your arms or hands.

Hand and Wrist Exercises

A good place to do hand exercises is at a table that supports your forearms. Do them after washing dishes, after bathing, or when taking a break from working with your hands. Your hands are warmer and more limber at these times.

3. Thumb Walk

Holding your wrist straight, form the letter "O" by lightly touching your thumb to each fingertip. After each "O," straighten and spread your fingers. Use the other hand to help if needed.

Shoulder Exercises

4. Good Morning Stretch

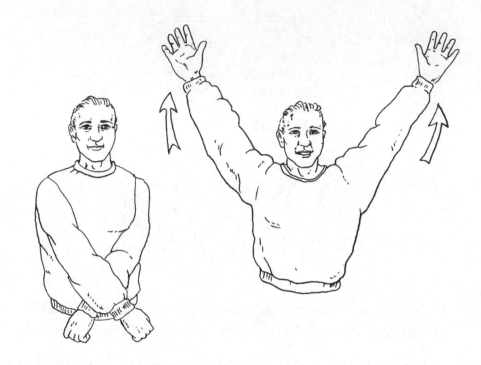

Start with hands in gentle fists, palms turned away from you, and wrists crossed. Breathe in and extend fingers while you uncross your arms and reach up as high as you can. Breathe out and relax.

5. Stave Exercise

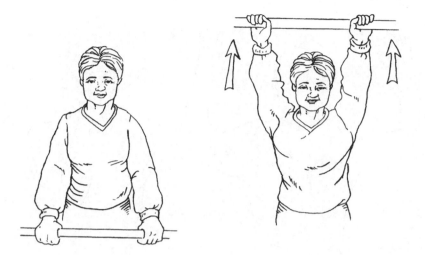

If one or both of your shoulders are tight or weak, you may want to give yourself a "helping hand." This shoulder exercise and the next allow the arms to help each other.

Use a walking stick, garden cane, or mop handle as your stave. Place one hand on each end and raise the staff as high overhead as possible. You might try this in front of the mirror. This stave exercise can be done standing, sitting, or lying down.

6. Pat and Reach

This double-duty exercise helps increase flexibility and strength for both shoulders. Raise one arm up over your head, and bend your elbow to pat yourself on the back. Move your other arm to your back, bend your elbow, and reach up toward the other hand. Can your fingertips touch? Relax and switch arm positions. Can you touch on that side? For most people, one position will work better than the other.

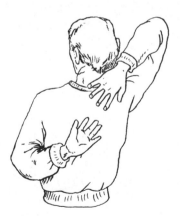

7. Shoulder Blade Pinch (VIP)

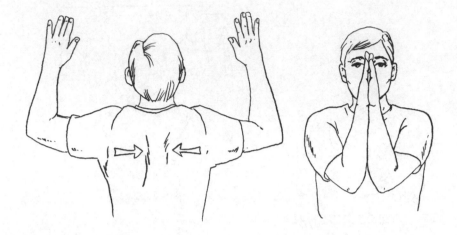

This is a good exercise to strengthen the middle and upper back and to stretch the chest. Sit or stand with your head in heads-up position (Exercise 1) and your shoulders relaxed. Raise your arms out to the sides with elbows bent. Pinch your shoulder blades together by moving your elbows as far back as you can. Hold briefly, then slowly move your arms forward to touch elbows. If this position is uncomfortable, lower your arms or rest your hands on your shoulders.

Back and Abdominal Exercises

8. Knee to Chest Stretch

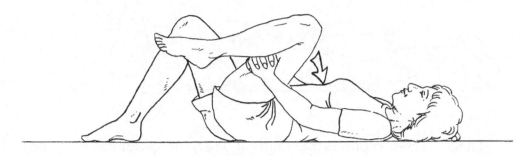

For a low back stretch, lie on the floor with knees bent and feet flat. Bring one knee toward your chest, using your hands to help. Hold your knee near your chest for 10 seconds and lower the leg slowly. Repeat with the other knee. You can also tuck both legs at the same time if you wish. Relax and enjoy the stretch.

9. Pelvic Tilt *(VIP)*

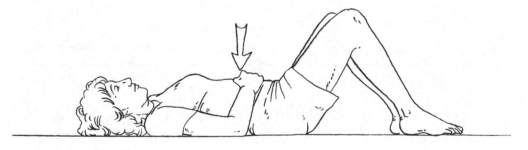

This is an excellent exercise for the low back. Lie on your back with knees bent, feet flat. Place your hands on your abdomen. Flatten the small of your back against the floor by tightening your stomach muscles and your buttocks. It helps to imagine bringing your pubic bone to your chin, or trying to pull your tummy in enough to zip up a tight pair of trousers. Hold the tilt for 5 to 10 seconds. Relax. Arch your back slightly. Relax and repeat the Pelvic Tilt. Keep breathing. Count the seconds out loud. Once you've mastered the Pelvic Tilt lying down, practise it sitting, standing, and walking.

10. Back Lift (VIP)

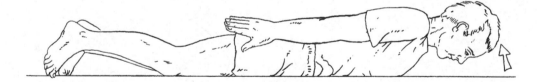

a. This exercise improves flexibility along your spine. Lie on your stomach and rise up onto your forearms. Keep your back relaxed, and keep your stomach and hips down. If this is comfortable, straighten your elbows. Breathe naturally and relax for at least 10 seconds. If you have moderate to severe low back pain, do not do this exercise unless it has been specifically prescribed for you.

b. To strengthen back muscles, lie on your stomach with your arms

at your side or overhead. Lift your head, shoulders, and arms. Do *not* look up. Keep looking down with your chin tucked in. Count out loud as you hold for a count of 10. Relax. You can also lift your legs, instead of your head and shoulders, off the floor.

Lifting both ends of your body at once is a fairly strenuous exercise. It may not be helpful for a person with back pain.

11. Low Back Rock and Roll

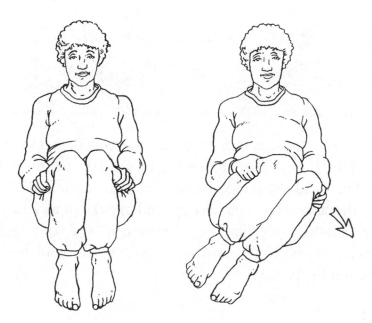

Lie on your back and pull your knees up to your chest with your hands behind the thighs. Rest in this position for 10 seconds, then gently roll knees from one side to the other, rocking your hips back and forth. Keep your upper back and shoulders flat on the ground.

12. Curl-Up

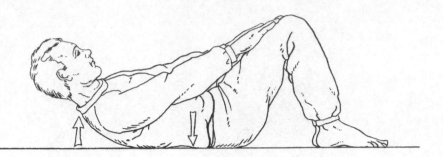

A curl-up, as shown here, is a good way to strengthen abdominal muscles. Lie on your back, *knees bent,* feet flat. Do the Pelvic Tilt (Exercise 9). Slowly curl up to raise your head and shoulders. Uncurl back down, or hold for 10 seconds and slowly lower. Breathe out as you curl up, and breathe in as you go back down. Do *not* hold your breath. If you have neck problems, or if your neck hurts when you do this exercise, try the next one instead. *Never* tuck your feet under a chair or have someone hold your feet!

13. Roll-Out

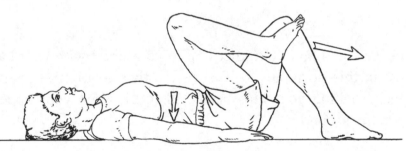

This is another good abdominal strengthener, and easy on the neck. Use it instead of the curl-up, or, if neck pain is not a problem, do them both.

- Lie on your back with knees bent and feet flat. Do the Pelvic Tilt (Exercise 9), and hold your lower back firmly against the floor.
- Slowly and carefully, move one leg away from your chest as you straighten your knee. Move your leg out until you feel your lower back start to arch. When this happens, tuck your knee back to your chest. Reset your pelvic tilt and roll your leg out again. Breathe out as your leg rolls out. Do *not* hold your breath. Repeat with the other leg.

You are strengthening your abdominal muscles by holding your pelvic tilt against the weight of your leg. As you get stronger, you'll be able to straighten your legs out farther and move both legs together.

Hip and Leg Exercises

14. Straight Leg Raises

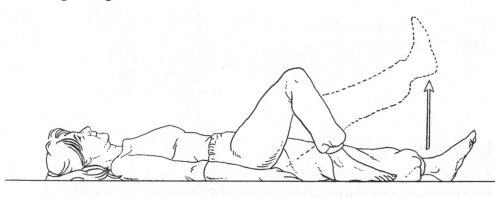

This exercise strengthens the muscles that bend the hip and straighten the knee. Lie on your back, knees bent, feet flat. Straighten one leg. Tighten the muscle on the top of that thigh, and straighten the knee as much as possible. Keeping the knee straight, raise your leg one to two feet (about 50 cm) off the ground. Do not arch your back. Hold your leg up and count out loud for 10 seconds. Relax. Repeat with the other leg.

15. Hip Hooray

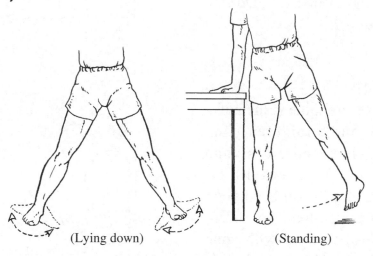

(Lying down)   (Standing)

This exercise can be done standing or lying on your back. If you lie down, spread your legs as far apart as possible. Roll your legs and feet out like a duck, then in to be pigeon-toed, move your legs back together. If you are standing, move one leg out to your side as far as you can. Lead out with the heel and in with the toes. Hold on to a worktop for support.

16. Back Kick *(VIP)*

This exercise increases the backward mobility and strength of your hip. Hold on to a worktop for support. Move the leg up and back, knee straight. Stand tall, and do not lean forward.

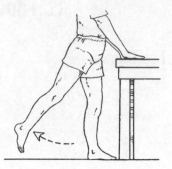

82

17. Knee Strengthener *(VIP)*

Strong knees are important for walking and standing comfortably. This exercise strengthens the knee. Sitting in a chair, straighten the knee by tightening up the muscle on top of your thigh. Place your hand on your thigh and feel the muscle work. If you wish, make circles with your toes. As your knee strengthens, see if you can build up to holding your leg out for 30 seconds. Count out loud. Do *not* hold your breath.

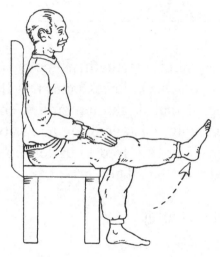

18. Power Knees

This exercise strengthens the muscles that bend and straighten your knee. Sit in a chair and cross your legs at the ankles. Your legs can be almost straight, or you can bend your knees as much as you like. Try several positions. Push forward with your back leg, and press backward with your front leg. Exert pressure evenly so that your legs do not move. Hold and count out loud for 10 seconds. Relax. Change leg positions. Be sure to keep breathing. Repeat.

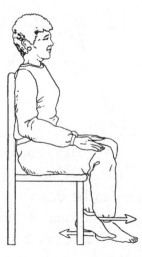

19. Ready-Go *(VIP)*

Stand with one leg slightly in front of the other in the position of having your heel on the floor ready to take a step with the front foot. Now tighten the muscles on the front of your thigh, making your knee firm and straight. Hold to count of 10. Relax. Repeat with the other leg.

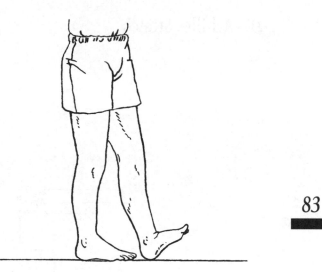

83

20. Hamstring Stretch

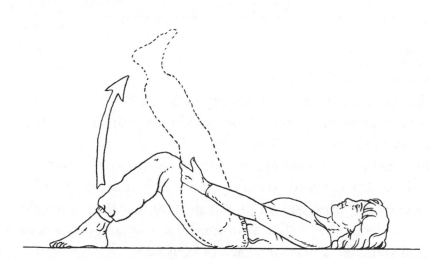

Do the self-test for hamstring tightness (page 88) to see if you need to do this exercise. If you have unstable knees, or "back knee" (a knee that curves backward when you stand up), do not do this exercise.

If you do have tight hamstrings, lie on your back, knees bent, feet flat. Grasp one leg at a time behind the thigh. Holding the leg out at arm's length, slowly straighten the knee. Hold the leg as straight as you can as you count to 10. You should feel a slight stretch at the back of your knee and thigh.

Be careful with this exercise. It's easy to overstretch and cause discomfort.

21. Achilles Stretch

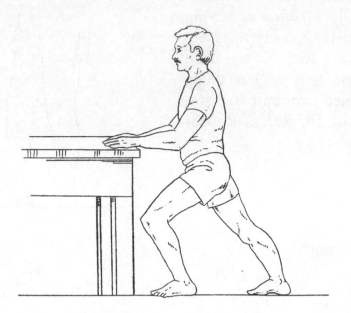

This exercise helps maintain flexibility in the Achilles tendon, the large tendon you feel at the back of your ankle. Good flexibility helps reduce the risk of injury, calf discomfort, and heel pain. The Achilles Stretch is especially helpful for cooling down after walking or cycling, and for people who get cramps in the calf muscles. If you have trouble with standing balance or muscle spasms, you can do a seated version of this exercise. Sit in a chair with feet flat on the floor. Keep your heel on the floor and slowly slide your foot (one foot at a time) back to bend your ankle and feel some tension on the back of your calf.

Stand at a worktop or against a wall. Place one foot in front of the other, toes pointing forward and heels on the ground. Lean forward, bend the knee of the forward leg, and keep the back knee straight, heel down. You will feel a good stretch in the calf. Hold the stretch for 10 seconds. Do *not* bounce. Move gently.

It's easy to become sore doing this exercise. If you've worn shoes with high heels for a long time, be particularly careful.

22. Tiptoes

This exercise will help strengthen your calf muscles and make walking, climbing stairs, and standing less tiring. It may also improve your balance. Hold on to a worktop or table for support and stand on your tiptoes. Hold for 10 seconds. Lower slowly. How high you go is not as important as keeping your balance and controlling your ankles. It is easier to do both legs at the same time. If your feet are too sore to do this standing, start doing it while sitting down. If this exercise makes your ankle jerk, leave it out, and talk to your physiotherapist about other ways to strengthen these calf muscles if needed.

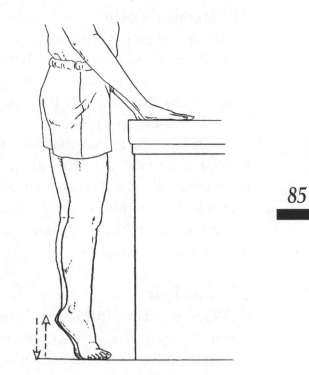

85

Ankle and Foot Exercises

Do these exercises sitting in a straight-backed chair with your feet bare. Have a bath towel and 10 marbles next to you. These exercises are for flexibility, strength, and comfort. This is a good time to examine your feet and toes for any signs of circulation or skin problems, and check your nails to see if they need trimming.

23. Towel Grabber

Spread a towel out in front of your chair. Place your feet on the towel, with your heels near the edge closest to you. Keep your heels down and your foot slightly raised. Scoot the towel back underneath your feet, by pulling it with your toes. When you have done as much as you can, reverse the toe motion and scoot the towel out again.

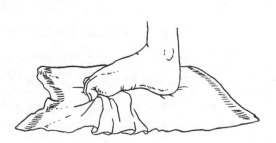

24. Marble Pick-Up

Do this exercise one foot at a time. Place several marbles on the floor between your feet. Keep your heel down, and pivot your toes toward the marbles. Pick up a marble with your toes, and pivot your foot to drop the marble as far as possible from where you picked it up. Repeat until all the marbles have been moved. Reverse the process and return all the marbles to the starting position. If marbles are difficult, try other objects, like dice or wads of paper.

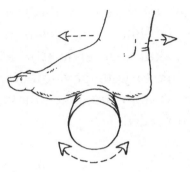

25. Foot Roll

Place a rolling pin (or a large dowel) under the arch of your foot, and roll it back and forth. It feels great and stretches the ligaments in the arch of the foot.

The Whole Body

26. The Stretcher

This exercise is a whole-body stretch to do lying on your back. Start the motion at your ankles as explained here, or reverse the process if you want to start with your arms first.

- Point your toes, and then pull your toes toward your nose. Relax.
- Bend your knees. Then flatten your knees and let them relax.
- Arch your back. Do the Pelvic Tilt. Relax.
- Breathe in, and stretch your arms above your head. Breathe out, and lower your arms. Relax.
- Stretch your right arm above your head, and stretch your left leg by pushing away with your heel. Hold for a count of 10. Switch to the other side and repeat.

Self-Tests

Whatever our goals, we all need to see that our efforts make a difference. Since an exercise programme produces gradual change, it's often hard to tell if the programme is working and to recognise improvement. Choose several of these flexibility and strength tests to measure your progress. Not everyone will be able to do all the tests. Choose those that work best for you. Perform each test before you start your exercise programme, and record the results. After every four weeks, do the tests again and check your improvement.

1. Arm Flexibility

Do Exercise 6 (Pat and Reach) for both sides of the body. Ask someone to measure the distance between your fingertips.

Goal: Less distance between your fingertips.

2. Shoulder Flexibility

Stand facing a wall, with your toes touching the wall. One arm at a time, reach up the wall in front of you. Hold a pencil, or have someone mark how far you reached. Also do this sideways, standing about three inches (8 cm) away from the wall.

Goal: To reach higher.

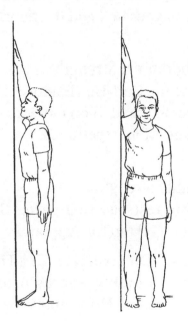

3. Hamstring Flexibility

Do the Hamstring Stretch (Exercise 20), one leg at a time. Keep your thigh perpendicular to your body. How much does your knee bend? How tight does the back of your leg feel?

Goal: Straighter knee and less tension in the back of the leg.

4. Ankle Flexibility

Sit in a chair with your bare feet flat on the floor and your knees bent at a 90-degree angle. Keep your heels on the floor. Raise your toes and the front of your foot. Ask someone to measure the distance between the ball of your foot and the floor.

Goal: One to two inches (3 to 5 cm) between your foot and the floor.

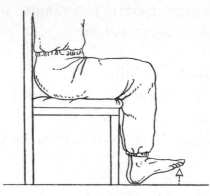

5. Abdominal Strength

Use the Curl-Up (Exercise 12). Count how many repetitions you can do before you get too tired to do more, or count how many you can do in one minute.

Goal: More repetitions.

6. Ankle Strength

This test has two parts. Stand at a table or worktop for support.

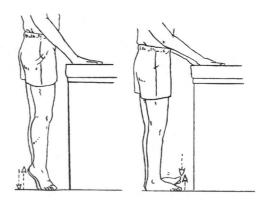

- Do Exercise 22 (Tiptoes) as quickly and as often as you can. How many can you do before you tire?

- Stand with your feet flat. Put most of your weight on one foot, and quickly tap the floor with the front part of your other foot. How many taps can you do before you tire?

Goal: Ten to fifteen repetitions of each movement.

• • •

Suggested Further Reading

Cooper, Kenneth H. *The Aerobics Program for Total Well-Being: Exercise, Diet, Emotional Balance*. New York: Bantam Doubleday, 1985.

Jerome, John. *The Pleasures of Staying Supple*. London: Souvenir Press, 2000.

Nelson, Miriam E. *Strong Women Stay Young*. New York: Bantam Books, 1998.

Torkelson, Charlene. *Get Fit While You Sit: Easy Workout From Your Chair*. Berkeley, Calif.: Hunter House Publishing, 1999.

89

CHAPTER
6

Exercising for Endurance:
Aerobic Activities

OW MUCH IS ENOUGH? One of the biggest problems with endurance (aerobic) exercise is that it is easy to overdo, even for those who don't have a chronic illness. Inexperienced and misinformed exercisers think they have to work very hard for exercise to do any good. Exhaustion, sore muscles, painful joints, and shortness of breath are the results of jumping in too hard and too fast. As a result, some people may discontinue their exercise programmes indefinitely, thinking that exercise is just not meant for them.

There is no magic formula for determining how much exercise you need. *The most important thing to remember is that some is better than none.* If you start slowly and increase your efforts gradually, it is likely that you will maintain your exercise programme as a lifelong habit. Generally it is better to begin your conditioning programme by underdoing rather than overdoing. Here are some rough guidelines to help you decide how much exercise is enough for you.

Several studies suggest that the *upper* limit of benefit is about 200 minutes of moderate-intensity aerobic exercise per week (see talk test below for what moderate intensity activity feels like). Doing more than that doesn't gain you much (and it increases your risk of injury). On the other hand, doing 100 minutes of exercise per week gets you about 90% of the gain, while 60 minutes of aerobic exercise per week yields about 75% of the gain. Sixty minutes is just 15 minutes of mild aerobic exercise four times a week!

Let's take a closer look at some general guidelines for the frequency, duration, and intensity of aerobic exercise. If you have a heart problem, check with your doctor before you start your exercise programme.

- *Frequency:* Five days a week is a good goal for aerobic exercise. Begin by taking every other day off to give your body a chance to rest and recover. We recommend that you rest at least one day per week.

- *Time:* Start with just a few minutes, and gradually increase the duration of your aerobic activity to about 30 minutes a session. Once this is achieved, you can gradually increase the intensity. For example, you could alternate intervals of brisk exercise with intervals of rest or easy exercise. For example, after 3–5 minutes of brisk walking, do 1–2 minutes of easy strolling, then another 3–5 minutes of brisk walking. Eventually, you can build up to 30 minutes of activity. Then gradually eliminate rest intervals until you can maintain 20–30 minutes of brisk exercise. If 30 minutes seems too long, consider two sessions of 10–15 minutes each. Either way appears to improve health significantly.

- *Intensity:* Safe and effective endurance exercise should be done at no more than *moderate intensity*. High-intensity exercise increases the risk of injury and causes discomfort, so not many people stick with it. Exercise intensity is measured by how hard you work. For a trained runner, completing a mile in 12 minutes is probably low-intensity exercise. For a person who hasn't exercised in a long time, a brisk 10-minute walk may be of moderate to high intensity. For others with severe physical limitations, 1 minute may be of moderate intensity. The trick, of course, is to work out what is moderate intensity for you. There are several easy ways to do this.

Talk Test

Talk to another person or yourself, sing, or recite poems out loud while you exercise. Moderate-intensity exercise allows you to speak comfortably. If you can't carry on a conversation or sing because you are breathing too hard or are short of breath, you're working too hard. Slow down. The talk test is an easy way to regulate exercise intensity.

If you have lung disease, the talk test might not work for you. If that is the case, try the perceived-exertion test.

Perceived Exertion

Another way to monitor intensity is to rate how hard you're working on a scale of 0 to 10. Zero, at the low end of the scale, is lying down, doing no work at all. Ten is equivalent to working as hard as possible, very hard work that you couldn't do longer than a few seconds. Of course, you never want to exercise as hard as that. A good level for your aerobic exercise routine is between 3 and 6 on this scale. At this level, you'll usually feel warmer, that you're breathing more deeply and faster than usual, that your heart is beating faster than normal, but you should not be feeling pain.

Remember, these are just rough guidelines on frequency, duration, and intensity, not a rigid prescription. Listen to your own body. Sometimes you need to tell yourself (and maybe others) that enough is enough. More exercise is not necessarily better, especially if it gives you more pain or discomfort. As *The Walking Magazine* said, "Go for the smiles, not the miles."

93

Heart Rate

Unless you're taking heart-regulating medicine (such as the beta-blocker propranolol), monitoring your heart rate while exercising is one way to measure exercise intensity. The faster the heart beats, the harder you're working. (Your heart also beats fast when you are frightened or nervous, but here we're talking about how your heart responds to physical activity.) Endurance exercise at moderate intensity raises your heart rate into a range between 60 and 80 percent of your safe maximum heart rate. Safe maximum heart rate declines with age, so your safe exercise heart rate gets lower as you get older. You can follow the general guidelines of Table 6.1, "Age–Exercise Heart Rate," or calculate your individual exercise heart rate. Either way, you need to know how to take your pulse.

Take your pulse by placing the tips of your middle three fingers at your wrist below the base of your thumb. Feel around in that spot until you feel the pulsations of blood pumping with each heartbeat. Count how many beats you feel in 15 seconds. Multiply this number by 4 to find out how fast your heart is beating in one minute. Start by taking your pulse whenever you think of it, and you'll soon learn the difference between your resting and exercise heart rates.

How to calculate your own exercise heart rate range:
1. Subtract your age from 220:
   Example: 220 – 60 = 160   You: 220 – _____ = _____
2. To find the *lower end* of your exercise heart rate range, multiply your answer in step 1 by [.6]:
   Example: 160 × .6 = 96   You: _____ × .6 = _____
3. To find the *upper end* of your exercise heart rate range, which you *should not exceed,* multiply your answer in step 1 by [.8]:
   Example: 160 × .8 = 128   You: _____ × .8 = _____

Table 6.1 *Age–Exercise Heart Rate*

Age Range	Exercise Pulse (15 sec)	Exercise Pulse (1 min)
0–30	29–39	116–156
30–40	28–37	112–148
40–50	26–35	104–140
50–60	25–33	100–132
60–70	23–31	92–124
70–80	22–29	88–116
80+	16–24	64–96

The exercise heart rate range in our example is from 96 to 128 beats per minute. What is yours?

Most people count their pulse for 15 seconds, not a whole minute. To find your 15-second pulse, divide both the lower-end and upper-end numbers by 4. The person in our example should be able to count between 24 (96 ÷ 4) and 32 (128 ÷ 4) beats in 15 seconds while exercising.

The most important reason for knowing your exercise heart rate range is so that you can learn not to exercise too vigorously. After you've done your warm-up and 5 minutes of endurance exercise, take your pulse. If it's *higher than the upper rate, don't panic*. Slow down a bit. Don't work so hard.

At first, some people have trouble keeping their heart rate within the "ideal" heart rate range. Don't worry about that. Keep exercising at the level with which you're most comfortable. As you get more experienced and stronger, you will gradually be able to do more vigorous exercise while keeping your heart rate within your "goal" range. But don't let the target heart rate monitoring become a burden. Recent studies have shown that even low-intensity exercise can provide significant health benefits. So use the "ideal" heart rate range as a rough guide, but don't worry if you can't reach the lower end of that range. The important thing is to keep exercising!

If you are taking medicine that regulates your heart rate, have trouble feeling your pulse, or think that keeping track of your heart rate is a bother, use one of the other methods to monitor your exercise intensity.

How Much Is Enough? The FIT Formula

The results of your aerobic exercise programme depend on how often you exercise (F = Frequency), how hard you work (I = Intensity), and how long you exercise each day (T = Time). In much the same way a doctor prescribes medicine to have a certain effect, you can select your own "exercise dose" to get the result you want. Your exercise dose comes from how you combine the frequency, intensity, and time of your exercise. A bigger dose gives you different benefits than a smaller dose.

- *Frequency:* Three to five days a week. Three days a week is the starting minimum. As you gain endurance and strength, you can do aerobic exercise more often. If you exercise more vigorously, 3 days is enough. If your aerobic exercise is a comfortably paced walk, you could build up to 5 or even 7 days a week.
- *Intensity:* No more than moderate intensity. Moderate intensity is being able to carry on a conversation while you exercise, a perceived-exertion level of no more than 6, or an exercise heart rate of no more than 75% of your age-predicted maximum heart rate.
- *Time:* Minimum of 30 minutes accumulated low to moderate physical activity. For health benefits, the activity may be accumulated in three 10-minute bouts during the day. To improve cardiovascular fitness, it may be necessary to exercise a bit longer each time.

People who are beginning an exercise programme should consider the following advice: **Adults should accumulate 30 minutes of moderate physical activity on most days of the week.** It is important to remember that this is a goal, not necessarily your starting point. If you can begin exercising just 2 minutes at a time, you are likely to be able to reach the recommendation of 10 minutes three times a day and achieve important health benefits.

When to Warm Up and Cool Down

Warm-Up

If you are going to exercise at an intensity that causes you to breathe harder or your heart to beat faster, it is important to warm up first. A warm-up means that you do at least 5 minutes of a low-intensity activity to allow your heart, lungs, and circulation to gradually increase their work. If you are going for a brisk walk, warm up with 5 minutes of slow walking first. If you are riding on an exercise bicycle, warm up with 5 minutes of no resistance and no more than 60 rpm (revolutions per minute). In an aerobic exercise class, you will warm up with a gentle routine before getting more vigorous. Warming up reduces the risk of injuries, soreness, and irregular heartbeats.

Cool Down

A cool-down period is important if you have exercised at an intensity that required you to breathe harder and your heart to beat faster, or if you felt warmer or perspired. Repeating the 5-minute warm-up activity or taking a slow walk helps your muscles gradually relax and your heart and breathing to slow down. Gentle stretching and flexibility exercises during the cool-down can be effective for increasing motion because your muscles and joints are warm and more easily stretched. Also, stretching gently now helps reduce the muscle soreness and stiffness that may follow vigorous exercise.

Endurance (Aerobic) Exercises

Many activities can be aerobic. We will examine in more detail a few of the more common ones, including walking, swimming, using an exercise bicycle, and low-impact aerobics.

Walking

Walking can condition your heart and lungs, strengthen bones and muscles, relieve tension, control weight, and generally make you feel good. Walking is easy, inexpensive, safe, and accessible. You can walk by yourself or with company, and you can take your exercise with you wherever you go. Walking is safer and puts less stress on the body than jogging or running. It's an especially good choice if you are older, have been sedentary, or have joint problems.

Most people with a chronic illness can walk as a fitness exercise. If you walk to the shops, to visit friends, and do household chores, then you'll probably be able to walk for exercise. Using a walking stick or walking aid need not stop you from getting into a walking routine. If you are in a wheelchair, use crutches, or experience more than mild discomfort when you walk a short distance, you should consider some other type of aerobic exercise, or consult a doctor or physiotherapist for help.

Be cautious the first two weeks of walking. If you haven't been doing much for a while, 10 minutes of walking may be enough. Build up your time with intervals of strolling. Each week increase the brisk walking interval by no more than 5 minutes until you are up to 20 or 30 minutes. Follow the frequency, duration, and intensity guidelines, and read these tips on walking before you start.

Walking Tips

Choose your ground. Walk on a flat, level surface. Walking on hills, uneven ground, soft earth, sand, or gravel is hard work and often leads to hip, knee, or foot pain. Fitness trails, shopping malls, school tracks, streets with pavements, and quiet neighbourhoods are good places to get started.

Always warm up and cool down with a stroll. It's important to walk slowly for 3 to 5 minutes to prepare your circulation and muscles for a brisk walk, and to finish up with the same slow walk to let your body slow down gradually. Experienced walkers know they can avoid shin and foot discomfort when they begin and end with a stroll.

Set your own pace. It takes practise to find the right walking speed. To find your speed, start walking slowly for a few minutes, then increase your speed to a pace that is slightly faster than normal for you. After 5 minutes, monitor your exercise intensity by checking your pulse, or using the perceived-exertion or talk methods. If you are above the range or feel out of breath, slow down. If you are below the range, try walking a little faster. Walk another 5 minutes and check your intensity again. If you are still below your exercise range, keep walking at a comfortable speed and simply check your intensity in the middle and at the end of each walk.

Increase your arm work. You can also raise your heart rate into the "ideal" or target exercise range by increasing arm work. (Remember that many people with lung disease may want to avoid arm exercises, since they can cause more shortness of breath than other exercises.) Bend your elbows a bit and swing your arms more vigorously. Alternatively, carry a one- or two-pound weight (.75 kg) in each hand. You can purchase hand weights for walking, hold a tin of food in each hand, or put sand, dried beans, or pennies in two small plastic bottles or socks. The extra work you do with your arms increases your intensity of exercise without forcing you to walk faster than you find comfortable.

Shoes

It's not necessary to spend a lot of money on shoes. Wear shoes of the correct length and width with shock-absorbing soles and insoles. Make sure they're big enough in the toe area: the "rule of thumb" is a thumb width between the end of your longest toe and the end of the shoe. You shouldn't feel pressure on the sides or tops of your toes. The heel counter should hold your heel firmly in the shoe when you walk.

Wear shoes with a continuous crepe or composite sole in good repair. Shoes with leather soles and a separate heel don't absorb shock as well as the newer athletic and casual shoes. Shoes with laces or Velcro let you adjust width as needed and give more support than slip-ons. If you have problems tying laces, consider Velcro closures or elastic shoelaces.

Many people like shoes with removable insoles that can be exchanged for more-shock-absorbing ones. Insoles are available in sporting goods stores and shoe stores. When you shop for insoles, take your walking shoes with you. Try on the shoe with the insole to make sure that there's still enough room inside for your foot to be comfortable. Insoles come in sizes and can be trimmed with scissors for a neat fit. If your toes take up extra room, try the three-quarter insoles that stop just short of your toes. If you have prescribed inserts in your shoes already, ask your doctor about insoles.

Possible Problems

If you have *pain around your shins* when you walk, you may not be spending enough time warming up. Try some ankle exercises before you start walking. Start your walk at a slow pace for at least 5 minutes. Keep your feet and toes relaxed.

Another common problem is *sore knees*. Fast walking puts stress on knee joints. To slow your speed and keep your heart rate up, try doing more work with your arms (see above). Do the Knee Strengthener and Ready-Go (Chapter 5, Exercises 17 and 19) in your warm-up to reduce knee pain.

Cramps in the calf and *heel pain* can be helped by doing the Achilles Stretch (Chapter 5, Exercise 21) before and after walking. A slow walk to warm up is also helpful. If you have circulatory problems in your legs, and experience cramps or pain in your calves while walking, alternate intervals of brisk and slow walking at whatever pace you can tolerate. Slow down and give your circulation a chance to catch up before the pain is so intense you have to stop. As you will see, such exercises may even help you to gradually walk farther with less cramping or pain. If this doesn't help, check with your doctor or physiotherapist for suggestions.

Maintain good posture. Remember the heads-up position in Chapter 5 and keep your shoulders relaxed to help reduce *neck and upper back discomfort*.

Swimming

Swimming is another good endurance exercise. The buoyancy of the water lets you move your joints through their full range of motion and strengthen your muscles and cardiovascular system with less stress than on land. Since swimming involves the arms, it can lead to excessive shortness of breath in people with lung disease. However, for people with asthma, swimming may be the preferred exercise as the moisture helps reduce shortness of breath. People with heart disease who have severely irregular heartbeats and have had a pace-maker permanently placed on their heart should avoid swimming. For most people with chronic illness, however, swimming is excellent exercise. It uses the whole body. If you haven't been swimming for a while, consider a refresher course.

To make swimming an endurance exercise, you will eventually need to swim continuously for 20 minutes. Use the frequency, duration, and intensity guidelines set out at the beginning of this chapter to build up your endurance. Try different strokes, modifying them or changing strokes after each lap or two. This lets you exercise all joints and muscles without overtiring any one area.

Swimming Tips

The breast stroke and crawl normally require a lot of neck motion and may be uncomfortable if you have neck pain. To solve this problem, use a *mask and snorkel* so that you can breathe without twisting your neck.

Chlorine can be irritating to eyes. Consider a good pair of *goggles*. You can even have swimming goggles made in your lens prescription.

A *hot shower* or soak in a warm bath after your workout helps reduce stiffness and muscle soreness. Remember not to work too hard or get too tired. If you're sore for more than two hours, go easier next time.

Always swim where there are qualified lifeguards if possible, or with a friend. Never swim alone.

Aquacise

If you don't like to swim, or are uncomfortable learning swimming strokes, you can walk laps in the pool or join the millions who are "aquacising"—exercising in water.

Aquacise is comfortable, fun, and effective as a flexibility, strengthening, and aerobic activity. The buoyancy of the water takes weight off hips, knees, feet, and back. Because of this, exercise in water is generally better tolerated than walking in people who have pain in the hips, knees, feet, and back. Exercising in a pool allows you a degree of privacy in doing your own routine, since no one can see you much below shoulder level.

Getting Started

Joining a water exercise class with a good instructor is an excellent way of getting started. Many Arthritis Care branches offer water exercise programmes in local hydrotherapy pools.

If you have access to a pool and want to exercise on your own, there are many water-exercise books available. One we recommend is *Hydrorobics*, by Joseph A. Krasevec and Diane C. Grimes (Human Kinetics Publishers, 1985). It contains a lot of good ideas for exercise in the water.

Water temperature is always a topic when people talk about water exercise. The Arthritis Foundation (in the US) recommends a pool temperature of 84°F (29°C), with the surrounding air temperature in the same range. Except in warm climates, this means a heated pool. If you're just starting to aquacise, find a pool with these temperatures. If you can exercise more vigorously and don't have a condition known as Raynaud's phenomenon (a circulation problem described in the supplement on Arthritis) or other cold sensitivity, you can probably aquacise in cooler water. Many pools where people swim laps are about 80–83°F (27–28°C). It feels quite cool when you first get in, but starting off with water walking, jogging, or another whole-body exercise helps you warm up quickly.

The deeper the water you stand in, the less stress there is on joints; however, water above mid-chest can make it hard to keep your balance. You can let the water cover more of your body just by spreading your legs apart or bending your knees a bit.

Aquacise Tips

Wear something on your feet to protect them from rough pool floors (important for people with diabetes) and to provide traction in the pool and at the poolside. Choices vary from terry cloth slippers with rubber soles (they stretch in water, so buy a size smaller than your shoe size) to footgear especially designed for water exercise. Some styles have Velcro tape to make them easier to put on. Beach shoes with rubber soles and mesh tops also work well.

If you are sensitive to cold or have Raynaud's phenomenon, *wear a pair of disposable latex surgical gloves*. Boxes of gloves are available at most chemists. The water trapped and warmed inside the glove seems to insulate the hand. If your body gets cold in the water, wear a T-shirt and/or full-leg Lycra exercise tights for warmth.

If the pool does not have steps, and it is difficult for you to climb up and down a ladder, *suggest positioning a three-step kitchen stool* in the pool by the ladder rails. This is an inexpensive way to provide steps for easier entry and exit, and it is easy to remove and store when not needed.

Wearing a *flotation aid or life jacket* adds extra buoyancy, to take weight off hips, knees, and feet. This makes exercising more comfortable for these joints.

You can *regulate how hard you work* in the water by the way you move. To make the work easier, move slowly. Another way to regulate exercise intensity is to change how much water you push when you move. For example, when you move your arms back and forth in front of you under water, it is hard work if you hold your palms facing each other and clap. It is easier if you turn your palms down and slice your arms back and forth with only the narrow edge of your hands pushing against the water.

If you have asthma, exercising in water helps to avoid the worsening of asthma symptoms that occur during other types of exercise. This is probably due to the beneficial effect of water vapour on the lungs. Remember, though, that for many people with lung disease, exercises involving the arms can cause more shortness of breath than leg exercises. You may want to focus most of your aquacising, therefore, on exercises involving mainly the legs.

If you have had a stroke, or have another condition that may affect your strength and balance, make sure that you have someone to help you in and out of the pool. Finding a position close to the wall or staying close to a friend who can lend a hand if needed are ways to add to your safety and security. You may even wish to sit on a chair in fairly shallow water as you do water exercises. Ask the instructor to help you design the best exercise programme, equipment, and facilities for your specific needs.

Using an Exercise Bicycle

Exercise bicycles offer the fitness benefits of cycling without the outdoor hazards. They're preferable for people who don't have the flexibility, strength, or balance to be comfortable pedalling and steering on the road. Some people with paralysis of one of their legs or arms can use exercise bicycles with special attachments for their paralysed limb. Indoor use of exercise bicycles may also be preferable to outdoor cycling for people who live in a cold or hilly area.

The exercise bicycle is a particularly *good alternative exercise.* It doesn't put excess strain on your hips, knees, and feet, you can easily adjust how hard you work, and weather doesn't matter. Use the bicycle on days when you don't want to walk or do more vigorous exercise, or can't exercise outside.

Make it Interesting

The most common complaint about riding an exercise bike is that it's boring. If you cycle while watching television, reading, or listening to music, you can become fit without becoming bored. One woman keeps interested by mapping out tours of places she would like to visit and then charts her progress on the map as she rolls off the miles. Other people set their bicycle time for the half hour of soap opera or news that they watch every day. There are videocassettes of exotic bike

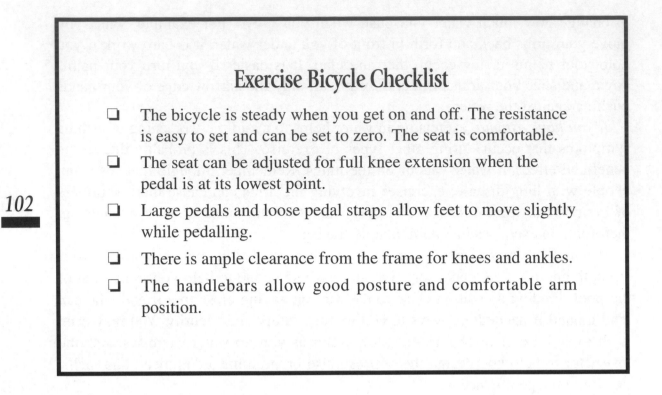

Exercise Bicycle Checklist

❏ The bicycle is steady when you get on and off. The resistance is easy to set and can be set to zero. The seat is comfortable.

❏ The seat can be adjusted for full knee extension when the pedal is at its lowest point.

❏ Large pedals and loose pedal straps allow feet to move slightly while pedalling.

❏ There is ample clearance from the frame for knees and ankles.

❏ The handlebars allow good posture and comfortable arm position.

tours that put you in the rider's perspective. Book racks that clip on to the handlebars make reading easy.

Cycling Tips

Cycling uses different muscles from walking. Until your leg muscles get used to pedalling, you may be able to cycle for only a few minutes. Start off with no resistance. Increase resistance slightly every two weeks. Increasing resistance has the same effect as cycling up hills. If you use too much resistance, your knees are likely to hurt, and you'll have to stop too soon before you get the benefit of endurance.

Pedal at a comfortable speed. For most people, 50–60 revolutions per minute (rpm) is a good place to start. Some bicycles tell you the rpm, or you can count the number of times your right foot reaches its lowest point in a minute. As you get used to cycling, you can increase your speed. However, faster is not necessarily better. Listening to music at the right tempo makes it easier to pedal at a consistent speed. Experience will tell you the best combination of speed and resistance.

Set your goal for *20 to 30 minutes of pedalling* at a comfortable speed. Build up your time by alternating intervals of brisk pedalling with less exertion. Use your heart rate, perceived exertion, or the talk test to make sure you aren't working too hard. If you're alone, try singing songs as you pedal. If you get out of breath, slow down.

Keep a record of the times and distances of your "bike trips." You'll be amazed at how much you can do.

On bad days, keep your exercise habit going by pedalling with no resistance, at fewer rpm, or for a shorter period of time.

Other Exercise Equipment

If you have trouble getting on or off an exercise bicycle, or don't have room for a bicycle where you live, you might try a restorator or arm crank. Ask your physiotherapist or doctor, or phone a medical supplier.

A *restorator* is a small piece of equipment with foot pedals which can be attached to the foot of a bed or placed on the floor in front of a chair. It allows you to exercise by pedalling. Resistance can be varied, and placement of the restorator lets you adjust for leg length and knee bend. A restorator can be a good alternative to an exercise bicycle for people who have problems with balance, weakness, or paralysis. People with other chronic illnesses, such as lung disease, may find the restorator to be an enjoyable first step in getting an exercise programme started.

Arm cranks are bicycles for the arms. They are mounted on a table. People who are unable to use their legs for active exercise can improve their cardiovascular fitness and upper-body strength by using the arm crank. It's important to work closely with a physiotherapist to set up your programme, because using only your arms for endurance exercise requires different intensity monitoring than using the bigger leg muscles. As mentioned previously, many people with lung disease may find arm exercises to be less enjoyable than leg exercises since they may experience shortness of breath.

There is a wide variety of exercise equipment in addition to what we've mentioned so far. These include treadmills, self-powered and motor-driven rowing machines, cross-country skiing machines, mini-trampolines, and stair-climbing machines. Most are available in both commercial and home models. If you're thinking about exercise equipment, have your objectives clearly in mind. For cardiovascular fitness and endurance, you want equipment that will help you exercise as much of your body at one time as possible. The motion should be rhythmical, repetitive, and continuous. The equipment should be comfortable, safe, and not stressful on joints. If you're interested in a new piece of equipment, if possible try it out for a week or two before buying it.

Exercise equipment that requires you to use *weights* usually does not improve cardiovascular fitness unless individualised "circuit training" can be designed. A weight-lifting programme alone builds strength, but it can put excessive stress on joints, muscles, tendons, and ligaments. Most people will find that the flexibility and strengthening exercises in this book will help them safely achieve significant increases in strength as well as flexibility. Be sure that you consult your doctor or physiotherapist if you prefer to add strengthening exercises involving weights or weight machines to your programme.

Low-Impact Aerobics

Most people find *low-impact aerobic dance* an enjoyable and safe form of exercise. "Low impact" means that one foot is always on the floor and there is no jumping. However, low impact does not necessarily mean low intensity, nor do the low- impact routines protect all joints. If you participate in a low-impact aerobic class, you'll probably need to make some modifications based on your condition.

Getting Started

Start off by *letting the instructor know who you are,* that you may modify some movements to meet your needs, and that you may need to ask for advice. It's easier to start off with a newly formed class than it is to join an ongoing class. If you don't know people, try to make friends. Be open about why you may sometimes do things a little differently. You'll be more comfortable and may find others who also have special needs.

Most instructors use music or count to a specific beat and do a set number of repetitions. You may find that the movement is too fast or that you don't want to do as many repetitions. *Modify the routine* by slowing down to half-time, or keep up with the beat until you start to tire and then slow down or stop. If the class is doing an exercise that involves arms and legs and you get tired, try resting your arms and do only the leg movements, or just walk in place until you are ready to go again. Most instructors will be able to instruct you in "chair aerobics" if you need some time off your feet.

Some low-impact routines use a lot of *arm movements* done at or above shoulder level to raise heart rates. Remember that for people with lung disease, hypertension, or shoulder problems, too much arm exercise above shoulder level can worsen shortness of breath, increase blood pressure, or cause pain, respectively. Modify the exercise by lowering your arms or taking a rest break.

Being different from the group in a room walled with mirrors takes courage, conviction, and a sense of humour. The most important thing you can do for yourself is to *choose an instructor who encourages everyone to exercise at her or his own pace* and a class where people are friendly and having fun. Observe classes, speak to instructors, and participate in at least one class session before making any financial commitment.

Aerobic Studio Tips

Wear shoes. Many studios have cushioned floors and soft carpet that might tempt you to go barefoot. Don't! Shoes help protect the small joints and muscles in your feet and ankles by providing a firm, flat surface on which to stand.

Protect your knees. Stand with knees straight but relaxed. Many low-impact routines are done with bent, tensed knees and a lot of bobbing up and down. This can be painful and is unnecessarily stressful. Avoid this by remembering to keep your knees relaxed (aerobics instructors call this "soft" knees). Watch in the mirror to see that you keep the top of your head steady as you exercise. Don't bob up and down.

Don't overstretch. The beginning (warm-up) and end (cool-down) of the session will have stretching and strengthening exercises. Remember to stretch only as far as you comfortably can. Hold the position and don't bounce. If the stretch hurts, don't do it. Ask your instructor for a less stressful substitute, or choose one of your own.

Change movements. Do this often enough so that you don't get sore muscles or joints. It's normal to feel some new sensations in your muscles and around your joints when you start a new exercise programme. However, if you feel discomfort doing the same movement for some time, change movements or stop for a while and rest.

Other kinds of exercise. Many exercise facilities have a variety of exercise opportunities: equipment rooms with cardiovascular machines, pools, and aerobic studios. If you have trouble with an hour-long aerobic class, see if you can join the class for the warm-up and cool-down and use an exercise bicycle or treadmill for your aerobic portion. Many people have found that this routine gives them the benefits of both an individualised programme and group exercise.

Self-Tests for Endurance/Aerobic Fitness

For some people, just the feelings of increased endurance and well-being are enough to demonstrate progress. Others may find it helpful to demonstrate that their exercise programme is making a measurable difference. You may wish to try one or both of these endurance/aerobic fitness tests before you start your exercise programme. Not everyone will be able to do both tests, so pick one that works best for you. Record your results. After four weeks of exercise, do the test again and check your improvement. Measure yourself again after four more weeks.

Distance Test

Find a place to walk, cycle, swim, or water-walk where you can measure distance. A running track works well. On a street you can measure distance with a car. An exercise bicycle with an odometer provides the equivalent measurement. If you plan on swimming or water walking, you can count lengths of the pool.

After a warm-up, note your starting point and cycle, or swim, or walk as briskly as you *comfortably* can for 5 minutes. Try to move at a steady pace for the full time. At the end of 5 minutes, mark your spot or note the distance or laps and immediately take your pulse and rate your perceived exertion from 0 to 10. Continue at a slow pace for 3 to 5 more minutes to cool down. Record the distance, your heart rate, and your perceived exertion.

Repeat the test after several weeks of exercise. There may be a change in as soon as four weeks. However, it often takes eight to twelve weeks to see improvement.

Goal: To cover more distance *or* to lower your heart rate *or* to lower your perceived exertion.

Time Test

Measure a given distance to walk, cycle, swim, or water-walk. Estimate how far you think you can go in 1 to 5 minutes. You can pick a number of blocks, actual distance, or lengths in a pool.

Spend 3 to 5 minutes warming up. Start timing and start moving steadily, briskly, and comfortably. At the finish, record how long it took you to cover your course, your heart rate, and your perceived exertion.

Repeat after several weeks of exercise. You may see changes in as soon as four weeks. However, it often takes eight to twelve weeks for a noticeable improvement.

Goal: To complete the course in less time *or* at a lower heart rate *or* at a lower perceived exertion.

Conclusion

Exercising to improve endurance has a central role in keeping our muscles and other systems 'conditioned'. When faced by the challenges of chronic disease the conditioned body is much better able to resist and overcome them.

• • •

Suggested Further Reading

Cooper, Kenneth H. *The Aerobics Programme for Total Well Being: Exercise, Diet, Emotional Balance.* London: Bantam, 1989.

Krasavec, Joseph, and Grimes, Diane C. *Hydrorobics: A Water Exercise Program for Individuals of All Ages and Fitness Levels.* Champaign, Ill.: Human Kinetics Publishers, 1985.

Stewart, Gordon W. *Active Living: The Miracle of Medicine for a Long and Healthy Life.* Champaign, Ill.: Human Kinetics Publishers, 1995.

Weddington, Michael. *Aerobic Sports Log: A Revolutionary Graphical Log Book for the Health-Conscious Individual.* Griffin Publishing,1997.

CHAPTER
7
Communicating

"**Y**OU JUST DON'T UNDERSTAND!**"** How often has this statement, expressed or unexpressed, summed up a frustrating verbal exchange? The goal in any communication between people is first that the other person understands what you are trying to say. Feeling you are not understood leads to frustration, and a prolonged feeling of frustration can lead to depression, anger, and helplessness. These are not good feelings for anyone, especially people with chronic illness. Dealing with a chronic illness can be frustrating enough, without adding communication problems.

Poor communication is the biggest factor in poor relationships, whether they be between spouses, partners, other family members or friends, co-workers, or doctors and patients. Even in casual relationships, poor communication causes frustration. How often have you been angry and frustrated as a customer, and how often is this because of poor communication?

When you have a chronic illness, good communication becomes a necessity. Your health care team, in particular, *must* "understand" you. As a self-manager, it is in your best interest to learn the skills necessary to make your communications as effective as possible.

In this chapter, we discuss ways to improve the communication process. Specifically, these are ways to express feelings in a positive way, how to ask for help, how to say "no," as well as how to best listen and how to get more information from the other person.

While reading this chapter, keep in mind that *communication is a two-way street*. As uncomfortable as you may feel about expressing your feelings and asking for help, the likelihood is that others are also feeling this way. It may be up to you to make sure the lines of communication are open. Be careful not to get caught in being uncomfortable with others because "they should know . . . ."

Expressing Your Feelings

Having a chronic condition brings about many feelings, some of them not pleasant. Here are some hints on how to express these feelings in a positive and constructive manner.

Start by taking a few moments to review exactly what the situation is that is bothering you and what you are feeling. For example, John and Steve had agreed to go together to a sporting event. When John came to pick up Steve, he was not ready and was not sure he wanted to go as he was having some trouble with his arthritic knees. The following conversation took place.

John: Why do you always spoil my plans? At least you could have phoned and I could have asked my son to go with me.

Steve: You just don't understand. If you had pain like I do, you wouldn't be so quick to criticise. You don't think of anyone but yourself.

John: Well, I can see that I should just go by myself.

In the above situation, neither John nor Steve had stopped to think about what was really bothering them or how they felt about it. Rather, they both blamed the other for an unfortunate situation.

The following is the same conversation in which both people were using thoughtful communications.

John: When we have made plans and then at the last minute you are not sure you can go, I feel frustrated and angry. I don't know what to do—go on without you, stay here and change our plans, or just not make future plans.

Steve: When this arthritis acts up at the last minute, I am also confused. I keep hoping I can go and so don't call you because I don't want to disappoint you and I really want to go. I keep hoping that my knees will get better as the day wears on.

John: I understand.

Steve: Let's go to the game. You can let me off at the gate before parking so I won't have to walk as far. Then I can take the steps slowly and be in our seats when you arrive. I do want us to keep making plans. In the future, I will let you know sooner if I think my arthritis is acting up.

John: Sounds good to me. I really do like your company and also knowing how I can help. It is just that being taken by surprise makes me angry.

John and Steve talked about the specific situation and how they felt about it. Neither blamed the other. Unfortunately, we are often in situations where the other person is using blaming communications or we are caught not listening and reverting to blaming communications. Even in this situation, thoughtful communication can be helpful. Look at the following example.

Jan: Why do you always spoil my plans? At least you could have phoned. I am really tired of trying to do anything with you.

Sandra: I understand. When this asthma acts up at the last minute, I am confused. I keep hoping I can go and so don't phone you because I don't want to disappoint you and I really want to go. I keep hoping that I will get better as the day wears on.

Jan: Well, I hope that in the future you will phone. I don't like being taken by surprise.

Sandra: I understand. If it is OK with you, let's go shopping now. I can walk a short way and rest in the coffee shop with my book while you continue to shop. I do want us to keep making plans. In the future, I will let you know sooner if I think my asthma is acting up.

In this last example, only Sandra is using thoughtful communication. Jan continues to blame. The outcome, however, is still positive with both people accomplishing what they want. The following are some suggestions for accomplishing good communications.

1. Always show regard for the other person. Avoid demeaning or blaming comments such as when Jan says, "Why do you always spoil my plans?" The use of the word "you" is a clue that your communication might be blaming.

2. Be clear. Describe a specific situation. For example, Sandra said, "When this asthma acts up at the last minute, I am confused. I keep hoping I can go and so don't phone you because I don't want to disappoint you and I really want to go. I keep hoping that I will get better as the day wears on."

3. Test your assumptions verbally. Jan did not do this. She assumed that Sandra was being rude by not phoning her. Remember that assumptions are often the place where good communications break down. One sign that you are making assumptions is when you are thinking "he or she should know . . . ."

112

4. Be open and honest about your feelings. Sandra did this when she talked about wanting to go, not wanting to disappoint Jan, and hoping that her asthma would get better.

5. Accept the feelings of others and try to understand them. This is not always easy. Sometimes you need to think about what has been said. Rather than answer immediately, remember that it is always acceptable to use "I understand" or "I don't fully understand. Could you explain some more?"

6. Be tactful and courteous. You can do this by avoiding sarcasm and blaming.

7. Work at using humour, but at the same time know when to be serious.

8. Be careful not to make yourself a victim by not expressing your needs and feelings and then expecting others to act the way you think they "should" act.

9. Finally, become a good listener.

"I" Messages

Many of us are uncomfortable expressing our feelings. This discomfort can be acute if doing so means we might seem critical of the person we're talking to.

Especially if emotions are high, attempts to express frustration can be laden with *"you" messages* that suggest blame. Its direction is toward the other person, causing the other person to feel as though he or she is under attack. Suddenly, the other person feels on the defensive, and protective barriers go up. The person trying to express feelings, in turn, feels greater anxiety when faced with these defensive barriers and the situation escalates to anger, frustration, and bad feelings.

CHAPTER 7 *Communicating*

The use of "I", however, doesn't strike out or blame. It is another form of communication that helps to express how *you* feel, rather than how the other person makes you feel. Here are some examples of *"I" messages:*

"You" message:	Why are *you* always late? We never get anywhere on time.
"I" message:	*I* get really upset when *I'm* late. It's important to *me* to be on time.
"You" message:	There's no way *you* can understand how bad I feel.
"I" message:	*I'm* not feeling well. *I* could really do with a little help today.

113

Watch out for *hidden* "you" messages. These are "you" messages with *"I feel . . ."* stuck in front of them. Here's an example:

"You" message:	*You* always walk too quickly.
HIDDEN *"You" message:*	*I feel* angry when *you* walk so quickly.
"I" message:	*I* find it difficult to walk quickly.

The trick to "I" messages is to avoid the use of the word *you,* and, instead, report your personal feelings using the word *I*. Of course, like any new skill, "I" messages take practice. Start by really listening, both to yourself and to others. Take some of the "you" messages you hear and turn them into "I" messages in your head. By playing this word game in your head, you'll be surprised at how quickly they become a habit in your own expressions.

There are some cautions to note when using "I" messages. First, they are not panaceas. Sometimes the listener has to have time to hear them. This is especially true if "you" messages and blaming have been the more usual ways of communicating. Even if at first using "I" messages seems ineffective, continue to use them and refine your skill.

Exercise—"I" Messages

Change the following statements into "I" messages. (Watch out for "hidden you" messages!)

You expect me to wait on you hand and foot!

Doctor, you never have enough time for me. You're always in a hurry.

You hardly ever touch me anymore. You haven't paid any attention to me since my heart attack.

You didn't tell me the side effects of all these drugs you're giving me or why I have to take them, doctor.

Also, some people may use "I" messages as a means of manipulation. If used in this way, problems can escalate. To be used effectively, "I" messages must report *honest* feelings.

One last note: "I" messages are an excellent way to express *positive* feelings and compliments! "*I* really appreciate the extra time you gave me today, doctor."

Asking for Help

Problems with communication around the subject of help are pretty common. For some reason, many people feel awkward about asking for help or in refusing help. Although this is probably a universal problem, it can come up more often for people with chronic illness.

It may be emotionally difficult for some of us to ask for needed help. Maybe it's difficult for us to admit to ourselves that we are unable to do things as easily as in the past. When this is the case, try to avoid hedging your request: "I'm sorry to have to ask this . . ." "I know this is asking a lot . . ." "I hate to ask this, but . . ." Hedging tends to put the other person on the defensive: "Oh no, what big favour is he about to ask of me?" Be specific about what help you are requesting. A general request can lead to misunderstanding, and the person can react negatively to insufficient information.

General request:	I know this is the last thing you want to do, but I need help to move. Will you help me?
Reaction:	Uh . . . well . . . I don't know. Um . . . can I get back to you after I check my other commitments? [probably next year!]
Specific request:	I'm moving next week, and I'd like to move my books and the contents of the kitchen beforehand. Would you mind helping me load and unload the boxes in my car on Saturday morning? I think it can be done in one trip.
Reaction:	I'm busy on Saturday morning, but I could give you a hand on Friday night, if you'd like.

People with chronic illness also sometimes deal with offers of help that are not needed or desired. In most cases, these offers come from people who are close to you and genuinely want to be helpful. A well-worded "I" message can refuse the help tactfully, without embarrassing the other person. "Thank you for being so thoughtful, but today I think I can handle it myself. I'd like to be able to take you up on your offer another time, though."

Saying "No"

Suppose, however, that you are the one being asked to help someone. Responding readily with "yes" or "no" may not be advisable. Often, we need more information before we can respond to the request.

If the request lacks enough information for us to respond, often our first feelings are negative. The example we just discussed about helping a person move is a good one. "Help me move" can mean anything from moving furniture up stairs to picking up the pizza for the hungry troops. Again, using skills that get at the specifics will aid the communication process. It is important to understand what the *specific* request is before responding. *Asking for more information or paraphrasing* the request will often help clarify the request, especially if prefaced by a phrase such as "Before I answer . . . " (this will hopefully prevent the person whose request you are paraphrasing from thinking that you are going to say yes).

Once you know what the specific request is and have decided to decline, it is important to *acknowledge the importance of the request* to the other person. In this way, the person will see that you are rejecting the *request,* rather than the *person.* Your turn-down should not be a put-down. "You know, that's a worthwhile project you're doing, but I think it's beyond my capabilities this week." Again, specifics are the key. Try to be clear about the conditions of your turn-down: will you always turn down this request, or is it just that there is a problem today or this week or right at this moment?

116 Listening

This is probably the most important communication skill. Most of us are much better at talking than we are at listening. We need to actually listen to what the other person is *saying and feeling.* Most of us are already preparing a response, instead of just listening. There are several levels involved in being a good listener.

1. *Listen to the words and tone of voice, and observe body language.* Sometimes it is difficult to begin a conversation if there is a problem. There may be times when the words being used don't tell you there is something bothering this person. Is the voice wavering? Does he or she appear to be struggling to find "the right words"? Do you notice body tension? Does he or she seem distracted? If you pick up on some of these signs, this person probably has more on her or his mind than words are expressing.

2. *Acknowledge having heard the other person.* Let the person know you heard them. This may be a simple "uh huh." On many occasions the only thing the other person wants is acknowledgment, or just someone to listen, because sometimes merely talking to a sympathetic listener is helpful.

3. *Acknowledge the content of the problem.* Let the other person know you heard both the content and emotional level of the problem. You can do this by restating the content of what you heard. For example: "You are planning a trip." Or you can respond by acknowledging the emotions: "That must be difficult," or "How sad you must feel." When you respond on an emotional level, the results are often startling. These responses tend to open the gates for more expression of feelings and thoughts. Responding to either the content or emotion can help communication along by discouraging the other person from simply repeating what has been said.

4. *Respond by seeking more information.* (See next section.) This is especially important if you are not completely clear about what is being said or what is wanted. There is more than one useful method for seeking and getting information.

Getting More Information

Getting more information from another person is a bit of an art, requiring special consideration. It can involve techniques that may be simple, or more subtle.

Ask for more. This is the simplest way to get more information. "Tell me more" will probably get you more, as will "I don't understand . . . please explain," "I would like to know more about . . . ," "Could you put that another way?" ,"How do you mean?", "I'm not sure I got that", and "Could you expand on that?"

Paraphrase. This is a good tool if you want to make sure you understand what the other person meant (not just what he/she *said*, but *meant*). Paraphrasing can either help or hinder effective communication, depending on the way the paraphrase is worded, though. It is important to remember to paraphrase in the form of a question, not a statement. For example, assume another person says:

> *Well, I don't know. I'm really not feeling up to par. This party will be crowded, there'll probably be smokers there, and I really don't know the hosts very well, anyway.*

If we were to paraphrase this as a *statement* rather than a question, it might look like this:

> *Obviously, you're telling me you don't want to go to the party.*

Paraphrased as a *question:*

> *Are you saying that you'd rather stay at home than go to the party?*

The response to the first paraphrase might be anger:

> *No, I didn't say that! If you're going to be that way, I'll definitely stay at home.*

Or the response might be no response . . . a total shutdown of the communication, because of either anger or despair ("He just doesn't understand."). People don't like to be told what they meant.

On the other hand, the response to the second paraphrase might be

> *That's not what I meant. I'm just feeling a little nervous about meeting new people. I'd appreciate it if you'd stay near me during the party. I'd feel better about it, and I might have a good time.*

As you can see, the second paraphrase promotes further communication, and you have discovered the real reason the person was expressing doubt about the party. You have gathered more information from the second paraphrase and no new information from the first one.

Be specific. If you want specific information, you must ask specific questions. We often automatically speak in generalities. For example:

Doctor: How have you been feeling?   *Patient:*   Not so good.

The doctor doesn't have much in the way of information about the patient's condition. "Not good" isn't very useful. Here's how the doctor gets more information:

Doctor: Are you still having those sharp pains in your left arm?   *Patient:*   Yes. A lot.

Doctor: How often?   *Patient:*   A couple of times a day.

Doctor: How long do they last?   *Patient:*   A long time.

Doctor: About how many minutes, would you say?

. . . and so on.

Doctors have been trained in ways to get specific information from patients, but most of us have not been trained to ask specific questions. Again, simply *asking for specifics* often works: "Can you be more specific about . . .?" "Are you thinking of something particular?" If you want to know "why", be specific about what it is. If you ask a specific question, you will be more likely to get a specific answer.

Simply asking *"Why?"* can unnecessarily prolong your attempt to get specific information. In addition to being a general rather than a specific word, "why" also makes a person think in terms of cause and effect, and he or she may respond at an entirely different level than you had in mind.

Most of us have had the experience where a three-year-old just keeps asking "Why?" over and over and over again, until the information the child wants is finally obtained (or the parent runs from the room, screaming). The poor parent doesn't have the faintest idea what the child has in mind and answers "Because . . ." in an increasingly specific order until the child's question is answered. Sometimes, however, the direction the answers take is entirely different than the child's question, and the child never gets the information he or she wanted. Rather than "why", begin your responses with "who", "which", "when", or "where". These words promote a specific response.

One last note about getting information: sometimes we do not get the correct information because we do not know what question to ask. For example, you may be seeking legal services from a Citizens' Advice Bureau. You phone and ask if they have a lawyer and hang up when the answer is no. If, instead, you had asked where you might get low-cost legal advice, you may have been given two or three contacts.

Communicating with Your Doctor

As a person with chronic illness, it is especially important to establish and maintain good communication with your doctor. The relationship you have with him/her must be looked on as a long-term one requiring regular work, much like a business partnership or a marriage.

Your doctor will probably know more intimate details about you than anyone except perhaps your spouse or partner or parents. You, in turn, should feel comfortable expressing your fears, asking questions that you may think are "stupid," and negotiating a treatment plan to satisfy you both, without feeling "put down" or that your doctor is not interested.

There are two things to keep in mind that will help to open, and keep open, the lines of communication with your doctor. How does the doctor feel? Too often, we expect our doctors to act as a warm-hearted computer—a gigantic brain, stuffed with knowledge about the human body, and especially *your* human body, able to analyse the situation and produce a diagnosis, prognosis, and treatment on demand—*and* be a warm, caring person who makes you feel as though you're the only person he or she cares about taking care of.

Actually, most doctors wish they were just that sort of person, but no doctor can be all things to all patients. They are human, too. They get headaches, they get tired, and they get sore feet. They have families who demand their time and attention, and they have to fight bureaucracies as formidable as the rest of us face.

Most doctors entered the gruelling medical training system because they wanted to make sick people well. It is frustrating for them not to be able to cure someone with a chronic disease like emphysema or arthritis. They must take their satisfaction from improvements rather than cures, or even in maintenance of existing conditions rather than declines. Undoubtedly, you have been frustrated, angry, or depressed from time to time about your illness, but bear in mind that your doctor has probably felt similar emotions about his or her inability to make you well. In this, you are truly partners.

120

Second, in this partnership between you and your doctor, *the biggest threat to a good relationship and good communication is **time***. If you or your doctor could have a fantasy about the best thing to happen in your relationship, it would probably involve more time for you both, more time to discuss things, more time to explain things, more time to explore options. When time is short, the anxiety it produces can bring about rushed messages, often "you" messages, and messages that are just plain misunderstood—with no time to correct them.

A doctor is usually on a very tight schedule. This fact becomes painfully obvious to you when you have had to wait in the doctor's office because of an emergency that has delayed your appointment. Doctors try to stay on schedule, and sometimes patients and doctors alike feel rushed as a consequence. One way to help you to get the most from your visit with the doctor is to take **P.A.R.T.**

| **Prepare** | **Ask** | **Repeat** | **Take action** |

Prepare

Before visiting or calling your doctor, *prepare your "agenda"*. What are the reasons for your visit? What do you expect from your doctor?

Take some time to make a written list of your concerns or questions. But be realistic. If you have 13 different problems, it isn't likely that your doctor can adequately deal with that many concerns in one visit. Identify your main concerns or problems. Writing them down also helps you remember them. Have you ever thought to yourself, after you walked out of the doctor's consulting room, "Why didn't I ask about . . . ?" or "I forgot to mention . . . ." Making a list beforehand helps you ensure your main concerns get addressed.

Mention your main concerns right at the beginning of the visit. Don't wait until the end of the appointment to bring up concerns, because there won't be the time to properly deal with them. Give your list to the doctor. If the list is long, expect that only two or three items will be addressed during this visit, and let your doctor know which items are the most important to you. Studies show that doctors allow an average of 18 seconds for the patient to state his or her concerns before interrupting with focused questioning. Preparing your questions in advance will help you use your 18 seconds well.

As an example of bringing up your concerns at the beginning of the visit, when the doctor asks, "What brings you in today?" you might say something like "I have a lot of things I want to discuss on this visit," *(looking at his or her watch and appointment schedule, the doctor immediately begins to feel anxious),* "but I know that we have a limited amount of time. The things that most concern me are my shoulder pain, my dizziness, and the side effects from one of the medicines I'm taking," *(the doctor feels relieved because the concerns are focused and potentially manageable within the appointment time available).*

Try to be as open as you can in sharing your thoughts, feelings, and fears. Remember, your doctor is not a mind reader. If you are worried, try to explain why: "I am worried that what I have may be contagious," or "My father had similar symptoms before he died," and so on. The more open you are, the more likely it is that your doctor can help you. If you have a problem, don't wait for the doctor to "discover" it. State your concern immediately. For example, "I am worried about this mole on my chest."

Give your doctor feedback. If you don't like the way you have been treated by the doctor or someone else on the health care team, let your doctor know. If you were unable to follow the doctor's advice or had problems with a treatment, tell your doctor, so that adjustments can be made. Also, most doctors appreciate compliments and positive feedback, but patients are often hesitant to praise their doctors. So, if you are pleased, remember to let your doctor know it.

Preparing for a visit involves more than just listing your concerns. You should be prepared to *concisely describe your symptoms to the doctor* (when they started, how long they last, where they are located, what makes them better or worse, whether you have had similar problems before, whether you have changed your diet, exercise, or medicines in a way that might contribute to the symptoms, etc.). If a treatment has been tried, you should be prepared to report the effect of the treatment. And if you have previous records or test results that might be relevant to your problems, bring them along. Be sure to tell your doctor about the trends (are you getting better or worse or are you the same?) and tempo (is it faster or slower?) of your problem, not just how you feel today. For example, "In general I am slowly getting better, although today I do not feel well." In treating a chronic condition, the trends and tempo are very important.

Ask

Another key to effective doctor-patient communication is asking questions. Getting comprehensible answers and information is one of the cornerstones of self-management. You need to be prepared to ask questions about diagnosis, tests, treatments, and follow-up.

1. *Diagnosis:* Ask your doctor what's wrong, what caused it, if it is contagious, what is the future outlook (or prognosis), and what can be done to prevent it in the future.

2. *Tests:* Ask your doctor if any medical tests are necessary, how they will affect your treatment, how accurate they are, and what is likely to happen if you are not tested. If you decide to have a test, find out how to prepare for the test and what it will be like.

3. *Treatments:* Ask about your treatment options including lifestyle change, medicines, surgery. Inquire about the risks and benefits of treatment and the consequences of not treating.

4. *Follow-up:* Find out if and when you should phone in or return for a follow-up visit. What symptoms should you watch for, and what should you do if they occur?

You may wish to take some notes on important points during the visit or consider bringing along someone else to act as a second listener. Another set of eyes and ears may help you later recall some of the details of the visit or instruction.

Repeat

It is extremely helpful to briefly repeat back to the doctor some of the key points from the visit and discussion. These might include diagnosis, prognosis, next steps, treatment actions, and so on. This is to double-check that you clearly understood the most important information. Repeating back also gives the doctor a chance to quickly correct any misunderstandings and miscommunications. If you don't understand or remember something the doctor said, admit that you need to go over it again. For example, you might say, "I'm pretty sure you told me some of this before, but I'm still confused about it." Don't be afraid too ask what you may consider a "stupid" question. These questions can often indicate an important concern or misunderstanding.

122

Take Action

When the visit is ending, you need to clearly understand what to do next. When appropriate, ask your doctor to write down instructions or recommend reading material for more information on a particular subject.

If, for some reason, you can't or won't follow the doctor's advice, let the doctor know. For example, "I didn't take the aspirin. It gives me stomach problems", or "I've tried to exercise before, but I can't seem to keep it up." If your doctor knows why you can't or won't follow advice, alternative suggestions can sometimes be made to help you overcome the barrier. If you don't explain the barriers to taking actions, it's difficult for your doctor to help.

123

Asking for a Second Opinion

Many people feel uncomfortable about asking their doctor for a second opinion about their diagnosis or treatment. Especially if you have had a long relationship with your doctor or simply *like* him or her, patients sometimes worry that asking for another opinion might be interpreted by the doctor as questioning his or her competence. It is a rare doctor whose feelings will be hurt by a sincere request for another opinion. If your condition is medically complicated or difficult, the doctor may have already consulted other doctors about your case, at least on an informal basis.

Even if your condition is not particularly complicated, asking for a second opinion is a perfectly acceptable, and often expected, request. Doctors prefer a straightforward request, and asking in a non-threatening "I" message will make this task simple:

> I'm *still feeling confused and uncomfortable about this treatment. I feel another opinion might help* me *feel more reassured. Can you suggest someone I could consult?*

In this way, you have expressed your own feelings without suggesting that the doctor is at fault. You have also confirmed your confidence in him or her by asking that he or she suggest the other doctor.

Good communication skills help make life easier for everyone, especially when chronic illness enters the picture. The skills briefly discussed in this chapter will hopefully help to smooth the communication process. In summary, the box on the next page gives examples of some words that can help or hinder.

Words That Help	Words That Hinder
At this moment, at this time, at this point, today	Never, always, every time, constantly
I	You
Who, which, where, when	Obviously . . .
How do you mean, please explain, tell me more, I don't understand	Why

124

Working with the Health and Social Care System

The National Health Service is going through many changes. This can lead to problems both for the patients as well as for the health and social care professionals. Your doctor or other care professionals may be just as upset as you when the system does not work well. New ways are being developed to get patients more involved in deciding how to make the NHS work better. If you are unhappy with the system, you can now do a lot more to help improve it. You can find out how local decisions are made and who makes them. Each Primary Care Trust (PCT) board has a patient representative. You can contact them by letter or phone and tell them about your concerns. If you have problems with your local GP surgery, you can contact the Practice Manager.

In every NHS hospital you now have the PALS (Patient Advocacy and Liaison Service) staff with whom you can discuss your problems. The new Commission for Public and Patient Involvement in Health (CPPIH) will soon begin to encourage active participation of the public in decisions affecting the NHS and the health and social care system more widely. Look out for opportunities in your area to contribute to this new agenda in active citizenship. The most important thing you can do is to work in partnership with your care professionals so that together you can find ways to make the system work well for you. You can also contact local Patients Forums or even become a member of a local Forum. Ask your local Expert Patients Programme Trainers for more information.

• • •

Suggested Further Reading

Beach, Wayne A. *Conversation About Illness: Family Preoccupations with Bulimia.* Hove, Sussex: Lawrence Erlbaum, 1996.

Beck, Aaron. *Love Is Never Enough: How Couples Can Overcome Misunderstandings, Resolve Conflicts, and Solve Relationship Problems Through Cognitive Therapy.* London: Harper Collins, 1989.

Egan, Gerard. *The Skilled Helper.* 7th Edition. Belmont, Cal.: Wadsworth, 2001.

Gabor, Don. *Talking with Confidence.* London: Sheldon Press, 1999.

Hargie, Owen. *A Handbook of Communication Skills.* 2nd Edition. London: Routledge, 1996.

Jones, J. Alfred, Gary L. Kreps, and Gerald M. Phillips. *Communicating with Your Doctor: Getting the Most out of Health Care.* Cresskill, N.J.: Hampton Press, 1995.

McKay, Matthew, Martha Davis, and Patrick Fanning.. *Messages: The Communication Skills Book.* Oakland, Calif.: New Harbinger Publications, 1983.

125

CHAPTER
8

Sex and Intimacy

COUPLES WHO LIVE WITH A CHRONIC HEALTH PROBLEM, with either one partner or both having a problem, face a challenge in keeping this important part of their relationship alive and well. Fear of injury or of bringing about a health emergency can dampen desire in one or both partners. Likewise, fear of increasing symptoms can frustrate couples, even if the symptoms occur only during sex itself. Sex, after all, is supposed to be joyful and pleasurable, not scary or uncomfortable!

For humans, sex is more than the act of sexual intercourse; it is also the sharing of physical and emotional sensuality. There is a special intimacy when we make love. Believe it or not, having a chronic health problem might actually improve your sex life by causing you to experiment with new types of physical and emotional stimulation for you and your partner. This process of exploring sensuality with your partner can open communication and strengthen your relationship as well. Additionally, natural "feel-good" hormones, called "endorphins," are released in our bloodstreams when we have sex.

For many people with chronic conditions, it is intercourse itself that is most difficult to sustain, because of the physical demands it places on our bodies. Intercourse brings about increased heart rate and breathing and can tax someone with limited energy or breathing or circulatory problems. Therefore, it is helpful to spend more time on sensuality or foreplay and less on actual intercourse. By concentrating on ways to arouse your partner and give pleasure while in a comfortable position, your intimate time together can last longer and be very satisfying. Many people enjoy climax without intercourse; others may wish to climax with intercourse. For some, climax may not be as important as sharing pleasure and they are satisfied without an orgasm. No matter how or if climax is reached, uncomfortable symptoms can be minimised if we concentrate on foreplay and sensuality rather than intercourse itself. There are many ways to enhance sensuality during sexual activity. In sex, as in most things, our minds and bodies are linked. By recognising this, we can increase the sexual pleasure we experience through both physical and cognitive stimulation.

Emotional concerns can also be a serious factor for someone with health problems. Someone who has had a heart attack or a stroke is often concerned that sexual activity will bring on another attack. People with breathing difficulties worry that sex is too strenuous and will bring on an attack of coughing and wheezing, or worse. Their partners may fear that sexual activity might cause these problems, or even death, and fear they would be responsible.

128

One of the most subtle and devastating barriers to fulfilling sexuality is the damage that has been caused to a person's self-image and self-esteem. Many report that they believe they are physically unattractive as a result of their disease—their paralysis, their shortness of breath, their weight gain from medicines, problems with their continence or the changing shape of their joints—a sense of not being a whole, functioning being. This causes them to avoid sexual situations, and they "try not to think about it." This often leads to depression, and depression leads to lack of interest in sex, and that leads to depression . . . a vicious cycle. Depression can be treated and you can feel better. For more on depression and how to help yourself overcome it, see Chapter 3 (page 39).

Even good sex can get better, though. Thankfully, there are ways you and your partner can explore sensuality and intimacy, as well as some ways to overcome fear during sex.

Overcoming Fear during Sex

Anyone who has experienced a chronic condition has experienced fear that it will get worse, or even that an episode could be life-threatening. Health problems can really get in the way of the activities that we want and need to do. When sex is the activity that fear affects, we have a difficult problem: not only are we denying ourselves an important, pleasurable part of life, but we probably feel guilty about denying our partner the same. Our partner may even feel more fearful and guilty than we do—afraid that he or she might hurt us during sex and guilty for maybe feeling resentful. This dynamic can cause serious problems in a relationship, and the stress and depression these problems cause can even cause more symptoms. We don't have to allow this to happen!

Remember the estate agents' maxim: "The three most important things to consider when buying a house are location, location, and location"? Well, for successful sexual relationships, the three most important things are (1) communication,

(2) communication, and (3) communication! The most effective way to address the fears of both partners is to confront them and find ways to alleviate them through effective communication and problem-solving. Without effective communication, learning new positions and ways to increase sensuality are not going to be enough. This is particularly important for people who may worry about how their health problem may make them look physically to others. Often, they find that their partner is far less concerned than they are.

When you and your partner are comfortable with talking about sex, you can go about finding solutions to the problems your chronic health problem imposes on you. To start with, you can share what kinds of physical stimulation you prefer and which positions you find most comfortable. Then you can share the fantasies you find most arousing. It's difficult to dwell on fears when your mind is occupied with a fantasy!

To get this process started, you and your partner may find some help with communication skills in Chapter 7 and problem-solving techniques in Chapter 1. Remember, if these techniques are new, give them time and practise. As we find with any new skill, it takes patience to learn to do them well.

Sensuality with Touch

The largest sensual organ of our bodies is the skin. It is rich with sensory nerves. The right touch on almost any area of our skin can be very erotic. Fortunately, sexual stimulation through touch can be done in just about any position. It can be further enhanced with the use of oils, flavored lotions, feathers, fur gloves—turn your imagination loose on this one! Just about any part of the skin can be an erogenous zone, but the most popular are the mouth (of course!), ear lobes, neck, breasts (for both sexes), navel area, hands (fingertips if you are giving pleasure, palms if you are receiving pleasure), wrists, small of the back, buttocks, toes, and insides of the thighs and arms. Experiment with the type of touch—some find a light touch arousing, others prefer a firm touch. It is not necessary to limit yourself to your hands, either. Many people become very aroused when touched with the lips, tongue, or sex toys.

Sensuality with Fantasy

What goes on in our minds can be extremely arousing. If it weren't, there would be no strip clubs, pornography, or even romantic novels. Most people engage in sexual fantasy at some time or another. There are probably as many sexual fantasies as there are people, and any are fine to mentally indulge in. If you discover a fantasy you and your partner share, you can play it out in bed, even if it is as simple as a particular saying you or your partner like to hear during sex. Engaging the mind during sexual activity can be every bit as arousing as the physical stimulation. It is also useful when symptoms during sex interfere with your enjoyment.

Overcoming Symptoms during Sex

130

Some people are unable to find a sexual position that is completely comfortable, or they find pain, shortness of breath, or fatigue during sex to be so distracting that it interferes with their enjoyment of sex or their ability to have an orgasm. This situation can pose some special problems. If you are unable to climax, you may feel resentful of your partner if he or she is able to climax, and your partner may feel guilty about it. If you avoid sex because you are frustrated, your partner may become resentful and you may feel guilty. Your self-esteem may suffer. Your relationship with your partner may suffer. Everything suffers.

One thing you can do to help deal with this situation is to time taking medication to be at peak effectiveness when you want to have sex. Of course, this would involve planning ahead! The type of medication may be important, too. If you take a narcotic-type painkiller, for example, or one containing muscle relaxants or tranquillisers, you may find that your sensory nerves are dulled along with your pain. Obviously, it would be counter-productive to dull the nerves that will give you pleasure. Your thinking may also be muddled due to the medication and make it more difficult to focus. Some medications can also make it difficult for a man to achieve an erection. Ask your doctor or pharmacist about possible timing or alternatives if this is a problem for you.

Another way to deal with uncomfortable symptoms is to become the world's best expert at fantasy! To be really good at something, you have to train for it, and this is no exception. The idea here is to develop one or more sexual fantasies that you can indulge in when needed, making it vivid in your mind. Then, during sex, you can call up your fantasy and concentrate on it. By concentrating on the fantasy, or on picturing you and your partner making love while you actually are, you are keeping your mind consumed with erotic thoughts rather than your symptoms. However, if you have not had experience in visualisation and imagery techniques, generally used for relaxation exercises such as those in Chapter 3, you will need to practise several times a week to learn it well. All of this practise need not be on your chosen sexual fantasy, however. You can start with any guided imagery tape or script such as the one in Chapter 3, working to make it more vivid each time you practise. Start with just picturing the images. When you get good at that, add and dwell on colours; then, in your mind, look down to your feet as you walk; then listen to the sounds around you; then concentrate on the smells and tastes in the image and feel your skin being touched by a breeze or mist; and, finally, feel yourself touch things in the image. Work on one of the senses at a time. Become good at one before going on to another. Once proficient at imagery, you can invest your own sexual fantasy and picture it, hear it, smell it, and feel it. You can even begin your fantasy by picturing yourself setting your symptoms aside. The possibilities are limited only by your imagination!

131

Learning to call on this level of concentration can also help you focus on the moment. Really focusing on your physical and emotional sensations during sex can be powerfully erotic. If your mind wanders (this is normal), gently bring it back to the here and now. ***IMPORTANT:*** *Do not try to overcome chest pain in this way. Chest pain should not be ignored, and a physician should be consulted right away.*

If you decide that you wish to abstain from sexual activity because of your chronic health problem, or if it is not an important part of your life, that's OK— but it is important to your relationship with your partner that he or she be in agreement with your decision. Good communication skills are essential in this situation, and you may even benefit from both of you discussing the situation with a professional therapist present. Someone trained to deal with important interpersonal situations can help facilitate the discussion.

Sexual Positions

In order to minimise symptoms during sex, as well as to minimise fear of pain or injury for both partners, it is important to find positions that are comfortable for both partners. Generally, comfortable positions can be found through experimentation. Everybody is different; no one position is good for everyone. We encourage you to experiment with different positions, possibly before you and your partner are too aroused for you to want to change to a more comfortable position. Experiment with placement of pillows or with using a sitting position on a chair.

No matter which position you try, it is often helpful to do some warm-up exercises before sex. Look at some of the stretching exercises from Chapter 5. Exercise can help your sex life in other ways, as well. Becoming more fit is an excellent way to increase comfort and endurance during sex. Walking, swimming, cycling, and so on, can benefit you in bed as well as anywhere else by reducing shortness of breath, fatigue, and pain. Also, learn your limits and pace yourself, just as you would with any other physical activity.

During sexual activity, it may be advisable to change positions periodically if your symptoms come on or increase when you stay in one position too long. This can also be done in a playful fashion, whereby it becomes fun for both of you instead of a chore. Stopping to rest is fine!

Other Considerations

It can be difficult to feel the urge for sex when you are in pain or are afraid that sex will cause you pain. If you have to overcome pain to become sexually aroused or to have an orgasm, it can be helpful to learn to focus on the moment or on a sexual fantasy. When you take your pain-relieving medicine, try to time it so that it works most effectively during sex. Find a comfortable position, take things slowly and easily, relax and take plenty of time to enjoy foreplay.

Your doctor is likely to know about solutions to any sexual problems caused by your condition. It may be possible to solve your problem by simply changing either your medicine or the time you take your medicine. Chronic health problems should not end sex. By talking with your partner and trying out new ideas, both the sex and your relationship can actually get better. There may be specific issues on sex related to your condition. These are dealt with separately in the disease-specific supplements to this handbook.

• • •

Suggested Further Reading

Association to Aid the Sexual and Personal Relationships of People with a Disability (SPOD), 286 Camden Road, London, N7 0BJ Tel 020 7607 8851. Contact for list of publications.

Ornstein, Robert, and David Sobel. *Healthy Pleasures*. Reading, Mass.: Addison-Wesley, Longman Inc., 1990.

Seidman, David. *The Longevity Sourcebook*. Los Angeles: Lowell House, 1997.

CHAPTER
9

Making Your Wishes Known

IT HAS BEEN SAID THAT LIFE IS THE GREATEST RISK FACTOR FOR DYING. All of us have feelings about our own death. Death may be feared, welcomed, accepted, or, all too often, pushed aside to be thought about at a different time. Somewhere, in the back of our minds, most of us have ideas about how and when we would like to die. For some of us, life is so important that we feel everything should be done to sustain it. For others, life is important only so long as we can be active participants. For many people, the issue isn't really death but, rather, dying. We have all heard about the eighty-year-old who died skiing. This may be considered a "good" death. On the other hand, we may have a friend or family member who spent years in a nursing home unaware of his or her surroundings. This is usually not what we would wish for ourselves.

While none of us can have absolute control over our own deaths, this, like the rest of our lives, is something we can help manage. That is, we can have input, make decisions, and probably add a great deal to the quality of our death. Proper management can lessen the negative impacts of our death on our survivors. This chapter deals with information to help you manage better some of the legal issues of death, specifically living wills and enduring power of attorney. Two good websites with information are www.growthhouse.org and www.ageconcern.

An enduring power of attorney is a document that *appoints another person to act on your behalf when you are incapable of doing so yourself.* It differs from a living will in two ways. First, a living will has effect when you are close to death while an enduring power of attorney is activated at such time you are incapable of acting on your own.

Secondly, a living will is not a legally binding document and acts as a guide to family, friends, and the health professionals as to what your wishes may be at this difficult time, whilst an enduring power of attorney has legal effect at a time you are incapable of acting yourself.

A general power of attorney allows you to appoint another person to act for you. For example, if you go on holiday while you are selling your house you may give your solicitor power of attorney to complete the sale on your behalf. An enduring power of attorney is a document in which you appoint someone else to act on your behalf concerning your legal and financial affairs. In other words, it allows someone else to make decisions for you, pay bills, even sell your home if you are unable to make decisions yourself (e.g., when in a coma or mentally incompetent). This document is activated only when for some reason you are unable to make decisions yourself.

134

One of the first things you need to do is decide whom you would like to work on your behalf. This can be your solicitor, friend, or member of the family. There are some considerations to be made in choosing who will act for you. This person should generally be available in the geographic area where you live. If he or she is not available to make decisions for you, he or she may not be much help. If you wish, you may name a second person to act for you if the primary person is not available. As a power of attorney gives someone so much control over your finance, it is advisable to draw it up with the advice of a solicitor.

Look for these characteristics in a person who you want to act on your behalf. It should be someone who:

- Is likely to be available should they need to act on your behalf
- Understands and respects your wishes and is willing to carry them out
- Is emotionally prepared and able to carry out your wishes
- Will not be emotionally burdened by carrying out your wishes

As you can see, finding the right person is a very important task. This may mean talking to several people. We will talk more about discussing your wishes with family, friends, and your doctor later. Lastly, ensure that people know where your enduring power of attorney and living will are kept.

For a living will, one of the most important things is deciding what you want to put in it. For example:

I do not want my life to be prolonged and I do not want life-sustaining treatment to be provided or continued

(1) If I am in an irreversible coma or persistent vegetative state; or (2) if I am terminally ill and the application of life-sustaining procedures would serve only to artificially delay the moment of my death; or (3) under any other circumstances where the burdens of the treatment outweigh the expected benefits. I want consideration to the relief of suffering and the quality as well as the extent of the possible extension of my life in making decisions concerning life-sustaining treatment.

I want my life to be prolonged and I want life-sustaining treatment to be provided unless I am in a coma or persistent vegetative state that my doctor reasonably believes to be irreversible. Once my doctor has reasonably concluded that I will remain unconscious for the rest, of my life, I do not want life-sustaining treatment to be provided or continued.

I want my life to be prolonged to the greatest extent possible without regard to my condition, the chances I have for recovery or the cost of the procedures.

Some charities provide forms on which you can write out any specific wishes. You are not required to give specific details but may wish to do so.

Knowing what details to write is a little complicated because none of us knows the exact circumstances that are likely to occur. However, you can get some idea by asking your doctor about what he/she thinks might be the most likely things to happen to someone with your condition. Your specific directions can discuss outcomes, specific circumstances, or both. If you discuss outcomes, then the statement should focus on what types of outcomes would be acceptable and which would not. For example, "resuscitate if I can continue to fully function mentally." The following are some of the more common specific circumstances that are encountered with major chronic diseases.

- Alzheimer's disease and other neurological problems are diseases that can leave you with little or no mental function. As we said earlier, these are generally not life-threatening, at least not for many years. However, things happen to these patients that can be life-threatening, such as pneumonia and heart attacks. What you need to do is decide how much treatment you want. For example, do you want antibiotics if you get pneumonia? Do you want to be resuscitated if your heart stops? Do you wish a feeding tube if you are unable to feed yourself? Remember, it is your choice as

135

to how you answer each of these questions. You may not want to be resuscitated but may want a feeding tube. If you want aggressive treatment, you may want to use all means to sustain life, or, more conservatively, you may not want any special means used to sustain life. For example, you may want to be fed but may not want to be placed on life support equipment.

- You have a very bad lung function that will not improve. Should you be unable to breathe on your own, do you want to be placed in an intensive care unit on mechanical ventilation (a breathing machine)? Remember, in this case you will not improve. To say that you never want ventilation is very different from saying that you don't want it if it is used to sustain life when no improvement is likely. Obviously, mechanical ventilation can be life-saving in cases such as a severe asthma attack when it is used for a short time until the body can regain its normal function. Here, the issue is not whether to use mechanical ventilation ever but rather, when or under what circumstances you wish it to be used.

- You have a heart condition that cannot be improved with angioplasty (cleaning out the arteries) or surgery. You are in the cardiac intensive care unit. If your heart stops functioning, do you want to be resuscitated? Like artificial ventilation, the question is not "Do you ever want to be resuscitated?" but, rather, "Under what conditions do you or do you not want resuscitation?"

From these examples it is hoped that you can begin to identify some of the directions that you might want to give in your living will. Again, to understand these better or to make them more personal to your own condition, you might want to talk with your doctor about what the common problems and decisions are for people like you.

In summary, there are several decisions you need to make when writing a living will.

- Generally, *how much treatment do you want?* This can range from the very aggressive, that is, doing many things to sustain life, to the very conservative, which is doing almost nothing to sustain life, except to keep you clean and comfortable.

- Given the types of life-threatening things that are likely to happen to people with your condition, *what sorts of treatment do you want and under what conditions?*

- If you become *mentally incapacitated,* what sorts of treatment do you want for *other illnesses* such as pneumonia?

Many people get this far. That is, they have thought through their wishes about dying and have even written them down in a living will. This is an excellent beginning but not the end of the job. A good manager has to do more than just write a note. He or she has to see that it gets acted on. If you really want your wishes carried out, it is important that you share them fully with your family, friends and your doctor. This is often not an easy task. In the following section, we will discuss ways to make these conversations easier.

Before you can have a conversation, all interested parties need to have copies of your living will. Once you have completed the documents, have them witnessed and signed. Make several copies. You will need copies for your, family members, and your doctor.

Now you are ready to talk about your wishes. Nobody likes to discuss their own death or that of a loved one. Therefore, it is not surprising that when you bring up this subject the response is often "Oh, don't think about that", or "That's a long time off", or "Don't be so morbid, you're not that sick." Unfortunately, this is usually enough to end the conversation. Your job as a good self-manager is to keep the conversation open. There are several ways to do this. First, plan on how you are going to begin your discussion of this subject. Here are some suggestions.

Prepare your living will, and then give copies to the appropriate family members or friends. Ask them to read it and then set a specific time to discuss it. If they give you one of those responses we talked about earlier, say that you understand this is a difficult topic, but that it is important to you that you discuss it with them. This is a good time to practice the 'I' messages discussed in Chapter 7. For example, "I understand that death is a difficult thing to talk about. However, it is very important to me that we have this discussion."

You might suggest that everybody makes out a living will and then share them. This could even be part of a family get-together. Present this as an important aspect of being a mature adult and family member. Making this a family project in which everyone is involved may make it easier to discuss. Besides, it will help to clarify everyone's values about the topics of death and dying.

If these two suggestions seem too difficult, or, for some reason, are impossible to carry out, you might *write a letter* or prepare an *audiotape* that can then be sent to members of your family. In the letter or tape, talk about why you feel your death is an important topic to discuss and that you want them to know your wishes. Then state your wishes, providing reasons for the choices you indicate. At the same time, send them a copy of your living will. Ask that they respond in some way or that you set aside some time to talk in person or on the phone with them.

This is not a topic that should be left to a mutual, unspoken understanding unless you don't mind if they decide differently from what you wish.

Talking with Your Doctor

From our research, we have learned that, in general, people have a much more difficult time talking to their doctors about their wishes surrounding death than to their families. In fact, only a very small percentage of people who have living wills ever share them with their doctor.

There are several reasons why it is important that this discussion take place. First, *you need to be sure that your doctor has values that are compatible with your wishes.* If you and your doctor do not have the same values, it may be difficult for him or her to carry out your wishes. Second, *your doctor needs to know what you want.* This allows him or her to take appropriate actions such as writing orders to resuscitate or not to use mechanical resuscitation should this be needed.

It is important to give your doctor a copy of your living will so that it can become a permanent part of your medical record. Again, the problem is often how to start this conversation with the doctor.

As surprising as it may seem, many doctors also find this a very difficult topic to discuss with their patients. After all, they are in the business of helping to keep people alive and well. They don't like to think about their patients dying.

If you wish, *plan a time with your doctor when you can discuss your wishes.* This should not be a side conversation at the end of a regular visit. Rather, start a visit by saying, "I want a few minutes to discuss with you my wishes in the event of a serious problem or impending death." When put in this way, most doctors will make time to talk with you. If the doctor says that he or she does not have enough time, then ask when you can make another appointment to talk with him or her

This is a situation in which you may need to be a little assertive. Sometimes a doctor, like your family members or friends, might say, "Oh, you don't have to worry about that, let me do it," or "We'll worry about that when the time comes." Again you will have to take the initiative, using an "I" message to communicate that this is important to you and you do not want to put off the discussion.

Sometimes doctors do not want to worry you. They think they are doing you a favor by not describing all the unpleasant things that might happen to you or the potential treatments in case of serious problems. You can help your doctor by telling him or her that having control and making some decisions about your future will ease your mind. Not knowing or not being clear on what will happen is more worrisome than being faced with the facts, unpleasant as they may be, and dealing with them.

Even knowing all of the above, it is still sometimes hard to talk with your doctor. Therefore, it might also be helpful to *bring someone* with you who is supportive of your wishes when you have this discussion. This person can facilitate the discussion and, at the same time, meet your doctor. This also gives everyone a chance to clarify any misunderstandings about your wishes. It opens the lines of communication so that if your family, friends and doctor have to act to carry out your wishes they can do so with few problems. If somehow you just "can't talk with your doctor", at least post him or her a copy of your living will to be placed in your medical records.

Now you have done all the important things. The hard work is over. However, remember that you can change your mind at any time. your wishes might change. Be sure to keep these documents updated. Like any legal document, it can be revoked or changed at any time. The decisions you make today are not forever

Making your wishes known about how you want to be treated in case of serious or life-threatening illness is one of the most important tasks of self-management. The best way to do this is to prepare a living will and share this with your family, close friends, and doctor.

A few more notes about preparing for death:

In most parts of the country hospice care is available. In everyone's life there comes a time when medical care is no longer helpful and we need to prepare for death. Today, we often have several weeks or months to make these preparations. This is when hospice care is so very useful. The aim of hospice care is to provide the terminally ill patient with the highest quality of life possible. At the same time, hospice professionals help the patient and the family prepare for death with dignity and also help the surviving family members. Some hospices are "in home" programmes. This means that the patient stays in his or her own home and the services come to them. In some places there are also residential hospices where people can go for their last days.

One of the problems with hospice care is that often people wait until the last few days before death to ask for this care. They somehow see asking for hospice care as "giving up." However, by refusing hospice care, they often put an unnecessary burden on themselves, friends, and family.

Hospice care can be most useful for the months before death. Most hospices only accept people who are expected to die within six months. This does not mean that you will be thrown out if you "outlive" your time. Six months is a guideline, not a fixed time. The message here is that if you, a family member, or a friend is in the ending stage of illness, find and make use of your local hospice. It is a wonderful final gift.

139

Choice In Dying
Hospital Hospice Own home

• • •

Suggested Further Reading

Cantor, Norman L. *Advance Directives and the Pursuit of Death With Dignity*. Bloomington, Ind.: Indiana University Press, 1993.

Elkington, J., and Hailes, J. *Manual 2000: Life Choices for the Future You Want*. Hodder and Stoughton, 1998.

Emanuel, Linda. "How Living Wills Can Help Doctors and Patients Talk About Dying: They Can Open the Door to a Positive, Caring Approach to Death." *British Medical Journal*, 320 (7250), pp. 1618-19, 17 June 2000. Discusses how living wills can be used positively to help prepare for death.

Molloy, W., and Mepham, V. *Let Me Decide: The Health Care Directive That Speaks for You When You Can't*. Penguin, 1993.

Patients Association, British Medical Association. *Advance Statements About Future Medical Treatment: A Guide for Patients*. Patients Association, 1997.

CHAPTER 10

Healthy Eating

DEVELOPING HEALTHY EATING HABITS is important for everyone. We know that a nutritionally balanced eating plan not only gives us more energy and endurance to be able to carry out our activities, but also makes us feel good and reduces our risk for certain health problems. While food alone cannot prevent or cure a chronic disease, learning to make healthier choices in the foods we eat can help us manage symptoms, prevent complications, and feel more in control of our health.

Changing our eating habits, however, is not easy. What we eat and how we prepare it are habits that have developed over years. For many of us, they are an important part of our family and cultural traditions. Therefore, suddenly trying to change everything about the way we eat is not only unrealistic, but unnecessary and unpleasant as well. If we want to make healthful changes in our eating habits that will last over time, and perhaps become the new practises we pass on to others, then these changes need to be small and gradual.

In this chapter, we offer some suggestions on how to begin making changes in our eating habits and how to enjoy doing it. We have included tips for planning well-balanced meals, making healthier food choices, managing a healthy weight, and minimising some of the problems commonly associated with eating and weight management. Just like any of the other self-management techniques discussed in this book, healthy eating will help you take control of your health.

What Is Healthy Eating?

Healthy eating does not mean that you can never eat your favourite foods again or that you have to "diet" or buy "special" foods. Rather it means learning to make healthier choices and eating in moderation. Eating is an important part of all our lives. Foods are chosen for all sorts of reasons, not just to get energy (calories) and nutrients. The taste, smell, colour, and appearance of food are all important. Cost, availability, and the way we live may also affect our food choices.

Sharing meals is also one of the ways we show and accept hospitality. For many of us, meals are an important part of our cultural and religious practice. So there are important skills to develop both in the choices we make and in communicating these choices to our friends.

A healthy, balanced diet can help you live a fitter, healthier life giving your body the resources it needs to resist the impact of chronic disease. Getting it right can reduce the risk of developing (or help manage) a range of health problems, including heart disease, diabetes, obesity, constipation, and tooth decay.

These are the simple guidelines for healthy eating:

- Enjoy your food
- Eat a variety of foods
- Eat plenty of foods rich in starch and fibre
- Eat plenty of fruit and vegetables
- Don't eat too much fat
- Don't eat sugary foods and drinks too often
- Eat foods that provide enough vitamins and minerals
- If you drink alcohol, drink sensibly
- Eat the right amount to be a healthy weight

If you are recovering from a serious illness and/or operation, your doctor may well recommend a particular diet that is designed for your own special needs and different to what is needed for a typical "healthy" diet. Speak to your doctor or dietitian if you have any concerns.

The Balance of Good Health

A balanced diet is one that includes a wide variety of foods, plenty of starchy foods and fruit and vegetables. Such a diet is demonstrated in Figure 10.1 on page 143.

Bread, Other Cereals, and Potatoes

Starchy foods should form the main part of your meals. This group includes bread, rolls, chapattis, breakfast cereals, oats, pasta, noodles, rice, potatoes, sweet

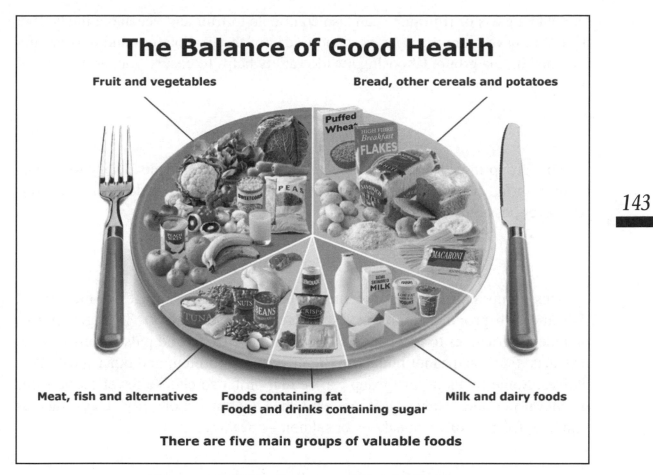

Figure 10.1 *The Balance of Good Health*

potatoes, plantains and green bananas, beans and lentils, and dishes made from maize, millet and cornmeal. This group does not include potato snacks, such as crisps.

The wholegrain varieties of starchy foods are a good source of fibre, for example wholemeal bread, brown rice, and wholegrain pasta. Baked beans are also a quick, cheap and tasty source of fibre. Choose lower fat methods of cooking foods in this group (such as boiling or baking rather than frying or roasting). If you have sauces, dressings or spreads with starchy foods, choose lower fat options.

Fruit and Vegetables

Try to eat at least five portions of fruit and vegetables each day. One portion is equivalent to a medium sized apple or banana, a bowl of salad or two serving spoonfuls of vegetables (or beans). This group includes all fresh, frozen and canned fruit as well as vegetables and salad vegetables. Beans and lentils, dried fruit and a glass of fruit juice can also contribute to fruit and vegetable intake (but try not to have more than one portion per day of these). Potatoes and nuts are not included in this group. Choosing a wide variety helps to ensure you are getting all the vitamins and minerals you need.

Milk and Dairy Foods

This group includes milk, cheese, yoghurt and fromage frais. Dairy foods can be high in fat, particularly saturated fat, so choose lower or reduced fat versions whenever possible.

Meat, Fish, and Alternatives

This group includes meat and meat products (such as sausages or meat pies), fish and fish products (such as fish fingers and fish cakes). This group also includes alternatives to meat and fish, such as eggs, beans and pulses, nuts and nut products, (such as peanut butter), textured vegetable protein and other meat alternatives. Some foods in this group can be high in fat so choose lower fat versions whenever possible. However, if you eat fish, eat a portion of "oily" fish – such as tinned or fresh sardines, mackerel or salmon – once a week.

Foods Containing Fat; Foods Containing Sugar

This group includes foods that can help to add taste, variety and enjoyment to the diet. There is no need to totally avoid them, but it is best to limit the amount eaten.

A small amount of fat is essential for health, but most of us eat far more than we need. "Foods containing fat" includes butter, margarine, low-fat spreads, cooking oils, mayonnaise and salad dressings. Use these foods sparingly and choose lower or reduced fat versions when possible.

"Foods containing sugar" includes, biscuits, cakes, puddings, ice-cream, chocolate, sweets, crisps, sugar, and sugar sweetened drinks. Try not to have these too often and when you do, have small amounts.

Choices That Improve Your Diet

How to Eat More Starchy Foods and Fibre

For most people, the move towards eating a healthier diet will mean eating more starchy foods. Starchy foods are low in fat and help to fill you up (particularly

PROTEINS are made from amino acids (the fundamental constituents of living matter) that are used by the body after being broken down when digested. Proteins are the building blocks for the enzymes and hormones that help regulate bodily functions. They are needed to maintain the body's immune system, which helps fight infection and build or repair damaged tissues. Proteins also provide energy for the body. Our bodies produce some proteins, but not all the ones it needs to carry out all functions. Therefore, we must get these proteins from the foods we eat. Meat, fish, poultry, eggs, and dairy products provide us with complete proteins. Vegetable sources of protein such as legumes, grains, nuts, and seeds are incomplete proteins; however, when eaten in the right combinations, vegetable sources can form complete proteins. Vegetable proteins provide additional health benefits because they are lower in fat and high in fibre and contain no cholesterol.

CARBOHYDRATES are the major source of energy for the body's muscles and metabolism. For this reason they should make up the majority of the foods and calories we eat each day. There are a variety of different foods that contain carbohydrates. These include starches, or complex carbohydrates, such as grains, rice, pasta, breads, legumes (peas and beans), root plants (potatoes, carrots, etc.), and other vegetables. Grains and vegetables also provide an excellent source of fibre. There are also simple carbohydrates, or sugars, which are found in fruits and some dairy products. These too are good sources of carbohydrate. Less desirable sources of carbohydrates include processed products or foods that are made with refined or table sugar, honey, syrups, and jellies; these sources provide calories but have little or no nutritional value.

FATS consist of substances called fatty acids and glycerol, which binds the fatty acids together. They can be saturated, monounsaturated, or polyunsaturated. Fats are used by the body for energy. While our bodies need some fat to help build, strengthen, and repair tissues, excess fat from the foods we eat is stored by the body, leading to weight gain and increased risk of heart disease. Meat, whole-milk dairy products, nuts, seeds, peanuts, and oils are rich sources of fat. Because fats contain twice the number of calories per gram than do proteins or carbohydrates, it is recommended we limit the amount of fat we eat, especially the saturated fats that come from animal sources or that are found in processed foods. Limiting foods that are high in saturated fat also helps to reduce dietary cholesterol, which is not a fat but tends to be present in high-fat dairy products, meats, and poultry.

VITAMINS AND MINERALS are necessary in small amounts to help build strong bones and muscles and to ensure that the body functions properly. They are found in varying amounts in the different foods we eat. Therefore, if we eat a variety of foods, the chances are we are getting the vitamins and minerals we need. Depending on our health needs, however, some people may need to take supplements, not to take the place of a balanced eating plan, but to help us reach the recommended daily allowance of certain vitamins and/or minerals. If supplements are needed, select one that contains 50–100% of the recommended daily allowance for the various vitamins and minerals. Examples include Centrum, Sanatogen, Haliborange, as well as the generic store brands. There is no need to take higher doses or "megadoses" of supplements unless prescribed and supervised by the doctor. Too much of some vitamins or minerals can create health problems and even some toxic reactions.

145

"wholegrain" or "high fibre" varieties). Starchy foods, such as potatoes, are often considered "fattening" but this is only true if they are cooked with fat or served with oils or other high fat foods. Therefore, it is best to choose boiled or baked potatoes over chipped or roast. Choose lower fat sauces (e.g. tomato based) to eat with rice and pasta. You can also change the amounts served — e.g. a little more pasta and a little less sauce.

How to Eat Less Fat

146

A small amount of fat in the diet is essential for our health, but most of us eat far too much. Eating too much fat, especially saturated fat, increases the risk of coronary heart disease. In particular, a high intake of saturated fat increases blood cholesterol levels, a risk factor for coronary heart disease. A diet high in fat will also be high in calories and you may gain weight. If you are overweight, cutting fat intake will be an important part of any weight reducing diet.

Some fats are easy to spot like cream, the fat on the outside of meat, butter and margarine. These are known as visible fats. There are also "hidden" fats in cakes, chocolate, biscuits, crisps, mayonnaise and pastry.

Examples of ways to reduce fat intake:

- Choose lower or reduced fat spreads (preferably high in mono- or polyunsaturates) and spread them more thinly.
- Try not using any spread sometimes, for example with beans on toast.
- Use semi-skimmed or skimmed milk.
- Try using low-fat yoghurt or low-fat fromage frais instead of cream, condensed or evaporated milk.
- Choose half-fat hard cheese or cottage cheese, or use a small amount of a very strong cheese, such as parmesan.
- Avoid oily salad dressings and mayonnaise. Make salad dressings with natural yoghurt, herbs, spices, tomato juice, vinegar or lemon instead.
- Cut down on crisps, chocolates, cakes, pastries and biscuits.
- Remove the skin from chicken, duck and turkey before cooking.
- Grill, microwave, steam, poach, bake or boil food rather than roasting or frying.
- Buy the leanest cuts of meat you can afford and trim off all the visible fat.

- Cut down on high fat meat products, such as, sausages and pies, and choose lower fat versions whenever possible.
- Use as little oil, margarine or butter for cooking as possible

How to Eat Less Sugar

Frequent consumption of foods containing sugar can contribute to tooth decay. In addition, if you are overweight, cutting back on sugar can help cut calories without losing any other nutrients.

Examples of ways to reduce sugar intake:

147

- Try drinking tea and coffee without sugar. You might find it easier to cut down a little at a time. If you find that you can't get used to drinks without any sweetness, try using one of the artificial sweeteners.
- Have chilled water (tap or bottled) rather than sweetened drinks.
- When buying canned soft drinks, try to choose low-calorie varieties.
- Use fresh, dried or canned fruit to sweeten breakfast cereals, cakes or puddings rather than using sugar.
- Buy fruit canned in natural, unsweetened juice rather than in syrup.
- Go easy on cakes, biscuits, burfi, sweet pastries, sweets and chocolate.
- Cut down on jam, marmalade, syrup, treacle and honey.
- Choose wholegrain breakfast cereals rather than those coated with sugar or honey.
- Use low-sugar varieties of any ready-made puddings and desserts you buy.
- Dried fruits contain high concentrations of sugar and can become stuck around the teeth, so avoid eating them frequently between meals.

How to Eat Less Salt

Salt is the main source of sodium in the diet. Most of us have more sodium in our diets than we need. Too much sodium in the diet can contribute to the development of high blood pressure. This in turn is a risk factor for coronary heart disease, kidney disease and strokes. In addition, for people that already have hypertension (high blood pressure), reducing their salt intake can help to reduce their blood pressure.

Examples of ways to eat less salt:

- Use less salt in cooking.
- Try to get out of the habit of adding salt to food at the table. Always taste food before you add salt.
- Flavour foods with lemon juice, herbs, spices, or vinegar instead of salt.
- Cut down on salty snack foods like crisps, salted nuts and other salty nibbles.
- When buying canned vegetables, choose the ones labelled 'no added salt'.
- Cut down on salted meats such as bacon, gammon and salt beef.
- Stock cubes are very salty. Try making your own stock or using fewer stock cubes but adding more herbs, garlic and spices for flavour.
- Many ready-prepared savoury dishes and sauces are very salty. Look at the label to find those with less added salt (or sodium) and monosodium glutamate.
- Limit sauces high in salt such as soy sauce.
- Salt substitutes can help reduce the amount of sodium in the diet — particularly if you miss the taste of salt. However, most salt substitutes still contain some salt. So, if you really want to lose the taste for salt, it is best to cut down the amount you use bit by bit, so you gradually lose the taste for it. Although you might miss the taste of salt at first you will soon discover subtleties of taste that were being obscured by the salt.
- There is little difference between sea salt and normal salt. As sea salt is often sold as crystals, you might end up eating more salt than you would using normal table salt.

Healthier Meals

Balance of Good Health (Figure 10.1, page 143) shows that you don't have to give up the foods you most enjoy for the sake of your health. It also stresses that a healthy diet is one based on a wide variety of foods and plenty of starchy foods, fruit and vegetables. A healthy diet also means enjoying the food you eat and not skipping meals, such as breakfast.

Everything you eat, including snacks as well as meals counts towards the balance of your diet. Many of the dishes we eat are a combination of foods from several of the food groups — like casseroles, spaghetti bolognaise, sandwiches and pizza. To make a healthier choice, it is important to think about how the main ingredients fit with the proportions shown in the Balance of Good Health.

Here are some suggestions of how to put healthy eating into practice, whether you are eating at home, at work, in a café or at a restaurant:

149

Breakfast

Bowl of porridge, cup of coffee — both with semi-skimmed milk — and a glass of unsweetened fruit juice. Using a lower fat milk helps to make this a good choice. You could add some fresh or dried fruit for a change and as an alternative to any added sugar or salt. A glass of fruit juice at breakfast counts towards your fruit and vegetable intake.

Bowl of cornflakes with sugar and whole milk. Improve this choice by using semi or skimmed milk. Increase the fibre content by choosing a "wholegrain", "wholewheat" or "high fibre" cereal. If you are particularly fond of cornflakes (or another lower fibre cereal), eat a higher fibre type every second day, or mix your favourite cereal with a higher fibre option. Try adding some fresh or dried fruit to sweeten your cereal rather than sugar.

White toast, butter and marmalade. Cup of tea with sugar. Using wholemeal bread for the toast would provide more fibre. Use a lower fat spread rather than butter or ordinary margarine. Allowing the toast to cool slightly before adding spread can help limit the amount you use. Try cutting down the sugar in your tea and go easy on the marmalade. You could try using fresh fruit — such as banana — rather than marmalade. Having a glass of fruit juice at breakfast would count towards your fruit and vegetable intake.

Main Meals

Spaghetti bolognaise — mincemeat, cooked with onion, carrots, celery, herbs, spices, tomato paste and tinned tomatos, and served with pasta. If you are cooking this meal from scratch, use lean mince (or skim the fat during cooking). Add more vegetables to the sauce than you would normally — such as extra tinned tomatoes and peppers (pimentos). You could also serve a little more spaghetti and a little less sauce than you would normally and have a side salad with the meal.

Roast chicken, roast potatoes, carrots and gravy. To reduce the fat content of this meal, have jacket or boiled potatoes instead of roast, if you make gravy from the pan juices, skim off the fat before serving. You can also remove the skin from the chicken. Add another portion of vegetables — either serve more carrots than you would normally, or serve an extra vegetable such as peas or cabbage.

150

Vegetable lasagne. If you are making this from scratch, cook plenty of vegetables in a minimum of oil. The white sauce can be high in fat, so try making it with cornflour and skimmed or semi-skimmed milk. If you add cheese to the sauce, use a half-fat variety or just a little strong, hard cheese (such as Parmesan or a very strong cheddar). Serve with extra vegetables or a side salad. For a more filling meal, you could also serve a bread roll.

Fish fingers, mashed potatoes, frozen mixed vegetables. Don't add too much butter or margarine to the mashed potatoes (or try it without any). To improve the flavour, add some chopped herbs instead. Grill or bake the fish fingers rather than frying them. Serve more vegetables than you would normally.

Puddings/Desserts

Fruit (fresh, tinned or dried) makes an excellent alternative to pudding. You can also add fruit to traditional choices, such as rice pudding or custard. Keep cakes and puddings for treats and special occasions, as they can be high in fat and calories. If you are making your own cakes or puddings, use lower fat ingredients whenever possible. For example, use semi or skimmed milk rather than whole, yoghurt or fromage frais instead of cream, fruit or sweeteners instead of sugar. It is also possible to buy lower or reduced fat cakes and puddings (though check the label — they may still be high in calories).

Ready-Prepared Meals

When buying pre-prepared meals, read the labels to select those that are lower in fat, sugar and salt. Most supermarkets now sell pre-prepared meals that are labelled as being healthier options. Remember that some common meals — beans on toast, vegetable based soups, microwaved baked potatoes — are also quick and healthy options.

Tips for serving pre-prepared meals:

- Have some vegetables with the meal—they can be quick to prepare if you use pre-washed, frozen or canned. Serve more than you would normally.
- Serve bread, rice, potatoes, pasta or pitta bread with the meal.
- Fresh, tinned or dried fruit, low-fat yoghurt or low-fat fromage frais are quick, ready-prepared desserts to try.
- Always follow the instructions on the package for any cooking or reheating that's involved.

151

Packed Lunches

Thinking of interesting and tasty packed lunches every day taxes anyone's imagination and can be difficult, especially when you're looking for healthier choices.

Examples of healthier options for packed lunches:

- Sandwiches made with thick-cut bread, rolls, crispbreads, muffins, chapattis and pitta breads
- Use fillings such as lean meat, chicken, boiled egg, mashed banana, cottage cheese, half-fat hard cheese, tuna, sardines, chopped raw vegetables, bean and nut spreads; avoid using fat spreads or mayonnaise in sandwiches in which you have a soft filling; if you do use spread, opt for a lower or reduced fat variety

Examples of other parts for a packed lunch:

- Pasta or rice salad — for example, pasta shells, pepper, cucumber chunks, cold chopped chicken, tuna or kidney beans
- Raw vegetables such as baby tomatoes or sticks of carrot and cucumber
- Soup, baked beans or tinned pasta in a wide-necked thermos flask with bread
- Raw vegetables such as sticks of carrot or celery, sweetcorn and salad vegetables
- Currant buns without icing, scones or teabreads
- Low-fat yoghurt or low-fat fromage frais
- Unsalted nuts (children under the age of five should not be given whole nuts due to the risk of choking)

152

Tips for Reducing Fat in Your Eating Plan

- Eat more poultry and fish, less red meat with a moderate size portion (2–3 oz, or 50–100 g, which is about the size of a deck of cards or the palm of your hand).

- Choose leaner cuts of meat.

- Trim off the outside fat and remove the skin from poultry.

- Eat egg yolks and organ meats (liver, kidneys, brains) in moderation.

- Broil, barbecue, or roast meats instead of frying them.

- Avoid deep-fried foods.

- Skim fat off stews and soups.

- Use low-fat or non-fat milk and milk products.

- Use added fats such as butter, margarine, oils, gravy, sauces, and salad dressings sparingly in food preparation (no more than 3–4 teaspoons [15–20 mL] per day).

- Use a non-stick pan with cooking oil spray.

Tips for Increasing Fibre in Your Eating Plan

- Build your meals around vegetbles, grain products, and fruits.

- Eat a variety of fruits and vegetables, raw or slightly cooked.

- Eat low-fat grain products such as whole-wheat breads, brown or whole-grain rice, and corn tortillas.

- Eat more beans and rice or lentils as meat substitutes.

- Snack on fruit or non-fat yogurt, not sweets, pastries, or ice cream.

- Drink plenty of water to help move the fibre through your system.

- Fresh fruit, such as apples, oranges, pears or peaches, or fruit canned in natural juice
- Dried fruit such as apricots or raisons

Snacks

All these ideas can make a healthier snack:

- Fresh fruit
- Vegetable based soups
- Pizza made on bread rolls or scone base with vegetables and a little half-fat hard cheese
- Sardines or baked beans on toast
- Wholegrain breakfast cereals, which are not sugar- or honey-coated, served with skimmed or semi-skimmed milk or eaten straight from the packet
- Plain popcorn sprinkled with paprika or Parmesan cheese
- Bread sticks, wholegrain crackers, crispbreads or rice-cakes with low-fat toppings
- Unsalted nuts

Eating Out and Take-Away Meals

Restaurant, cafe, and take-away meals are often convenient and tasty, but can be high in fat. You may be able to ask for your meal or snack to be prepared with less fat and more vegetables – just ask when you order. Remember that vegetarian options may not be automatically healthier if they are cooked with a lot of oil, cream and / or cheese.

Examples of healthier options include:

- Sandwiches with lower fat fillings
- Salads without dressing or with lower fat dressing (e.g. yogurt dressing)
- Baked potato without butter and with low-fat fillings such as cottage cheese, baked beans, ratatouille, chicken and mushroom, tuna (without mayonnaise) or chilli con carne
- Ask for burgers (beef, chicken, fish or bean) to be served in wholemeal buns with salad and skip the extra cheese and mayonnaise

- Choose thick cut rather than thin cut chips, go easy on the salt and if you want a sauce, opt for vinegar or ketchup rather than mayonnaise
- Avoid cream or cheese based sauces for meat, fish or pasta
- Shish kebabs in pitta bread with salad are a healthier option than donor kebabs
- Large helping of plain noodles or rice with stir-fried vegetables
- Tandoori chicken or chicken tikka with salad and chapattis or rice
- When ordering a pizza, ask for a little less cheese but extra vegetables
- When eating out, always have vegetables or salad with your meal, and go easy on the butter or dressing

Food Labels

Many food labels list the amount of calories and fat in the food. Before you buy foods and drinks, check the labels carefully. You will often find there is a healthier alternative available that doesn't cost any more — for example, lower in fat, containing less salt and/or sugar.

Some food labels make claims that the food has particular benefits. Specific claims like "low in calories" or "rich in vitamin C" have to meet legal conditions. Vague claims like "natural goodness" are meaningless from a health point of view. Many manufacturers and supermarkets use labels or symbols to identify foods that are lower in fat, sugar or salt, or higher in fibre. These can be useful as a quick guide, but if you are concerned about the content of foods, it is best to compare the food labels in detail. When a claim such as 'low-fat' is made, it is compulsory to give nutritional information on the label. Use the '100g' column to compare different products of similar kinds of foods and to choose the lower fat, sugar and salt (sodium) varieties.

Food Additives

Additives are added to food to help prolong its storage life, to make it easier to manufacture, to improve the flavour and to make it look more attractive to eat. Some additives are "natural" substances, for example salt, some colourings, vitamin C, and lecithin.

Additives are listed alongside ingredients on most packaged foods. Many additives are known by a European Union number (E number). All the additives with E numbers have been tested for safety. The amount of an additive that is added to individual foodstuffs is strictly controlled. A very small number of people are allergic to additives, and, indeed, to some ordinary food stuffs. For most people following a healthy diet, there is little need to be overly concerned about the additives present in food.

Managing a Healthy Weight

Food provides the energy (or calories) your body needs to sustain body processes, and for everyday physical activities such as walking, lifting and exercising. If the food you eat provides more energy than you require, the excess is converted into fat, and you will put on weight.

It is not healthy to be either underweight or overweight. If you don't eat enough food you may not be getting all the nutrients you need from your diet and you may become underweight, However, in Britain, more than 50 per cent of the population is overweight and has too much body fat.

A healthy weight is one whereby you reduce your risk of developing health problems, or further complicating existing ones, and feel better both mentally and physically. Finding a healthy weight depends on several factors, such as your age, your activity level, how much of your weight is fat, where the fat is on your body, and whether or not you have weight related problems such as high blood pressure or a family history of such problems. Achieving and/maintaining a healthy weight is important for everyone. Weight can have a considerable impact on your disease symptoms and your ability to exercise or otherwise mange health problems. For example, if you have diabetes, high blood pressure and/or high blood cholesterol, losing even a modest amount of weight will improve your symptoms.

For a rough guide whether you are a healthy weight, check your weight on the chart in Figure 10.2 (page 158).

Excess fat around your waist is particularly risky. A waist circumference of more than 94cm in men and more than 80cm in women is associated with an increased risk of heart disease and diabetes.

Speak to your doctor, nurse or dietitian about what is a healthy weight for you, given your condition and treatment needs. You may already be at a healthy weight and need only to maintain it by eating well and staying active. If you would benefit from losing some weight, they will be able to help you plan a suitable weight loss strategy.

Making small, acceptable alterations to your diet and lifestyle can result in a gradual, sustained weight loss. For most people, any suggested weight reducing diet will be in line with the Balance of Good Health (page 143) and the key aims will be to cut down on the amount of fat eaten (which is high in calories) and to increase the amount of starchy foods, fruit and vegetables.

People following a weight reducing diet may also be encouraged to watch the size of portions served, to eat regularly and not to skip meals. Walking more often, using the stairs instead of the lift, putting a bit more effort into housework and taking part in enjoyable activities such as golf or dancing are simple ways of being more active. Speak to your doctor about the best options for you.

156

Why Change My Weight?

The reasons for losing or gaining weight are different for each individual. The most obvious reason may be your physical health, but there may also be psychological or emotional reasons for wanting to change. Examine for yourself why you want to change.

For example, changing my weight will help me . . .

- Lessen my disease symptoms (e.g., pain, fatigue, shortness of breath, control blood sugar)
- Give me more energy to do the things I want to do
- Feel better about myself
- Change the way others perceive me
- Feel more in control of my disease and/or my life

If you have other reasons, jot them down here:

_____

_____

_____

The decision to change weight is a very personal one. To help you decide whether or not you are ready to make any changes, ask yourself the following questions:

What Will I Have to Change?

Two ingredients for successful weight management are developing an active lifestyle and making changes in your eating patterns. Let's look closely at what each of these involves.

An active lifestyle implies doing some physical activity that burns calories and regulates appetite and metabolism, both important for weight management.

Physical activity can also help you develop more strength and stamina, as well as move and breathe more easily. In other words, activity doesn't wear you down or out, but actually boosts your energy level. You will find much more information about exercise and tips for choosing activities that suit *your* needs and lifestyle in Chapters 4 to 6.

Making changes in your eating habits starts by making small, gradual changes in what you eat. This may mean changing the emphasis or quantity of certain foods you eat. You will find tips for doing this at the beginning of the chapter.

157

While most of us are concerned with losing weight and keeping it off, some people with chronic disease struggle to gain or maintain a healthy weight. If you experience a continual or extreme weight loss because your disease or treatment interferes with your appetite and/or depletes your body of valuable nutrients (such as protein, vitamins, and minerals), you may need to work at gaining weight.

Some common problems associated with making changes in your eating habits and/or weight management are discussed on pages 159-169.

You can also find more information on healthy eating in the references listed at the end of this chapter.

Am I Ready to Change for Good?

Success is important in weight management. Therefore, the next step is to evaluate whether or not you are ready to make these changes. If you are not ready, you may be setting yourself up for failure and those nasty weight "ups and downs." This is not only discouraging but unhealthy as well. For this reason it is helpful to plan ahead by considering the following types of questions.:

- Is there someone or something that will make it easier for you to change?
- Are there problems or obstacles that will keep you from becoming more active or changing the way you eat?
- Will worries or concerns about family, friends, work, or other commitments affect your ability to carry out your plans successfully at this time?

Looking ahead at these factors can help you find ways to build support for desired changes, as well as minimise possible problems you may encounter along the way. Use the accompanying chart (Figure 10.2) to help you identify some of these factors.

After you have examined these things, you may find that now is not the right time to start anything. If it is *not, set a date in the future* for a time when you will

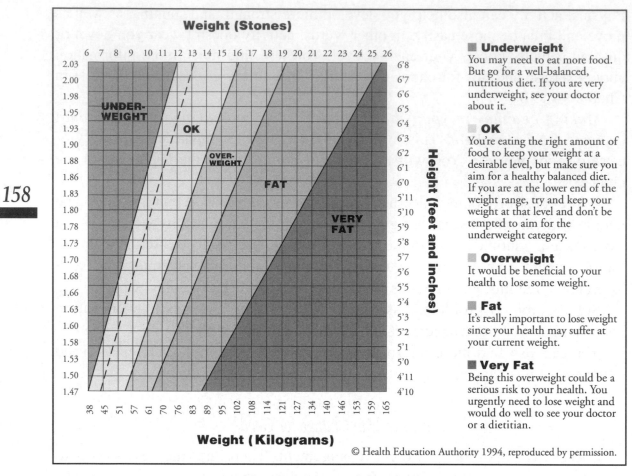

Weight (Stones)

UNDER-WEIGHT

OK

OVER-WEIGHT

FAT

VERY FAT

Height (feet and inches)

Weight (Kilograms)

■ **Underweight**
You may need to eat more food. But go for a well-balanced, nutritious diet. If you are very underweight, see your doctor about it.

■ **OK**
You're eating the right amount of food to keep your weight at a desirable level, but make sure you aim for a healthy balanced diet. If you are at the lower end of the weight range, try and keep your weight at that level and don't be tempted to aim for the underweight category.

■ **Overweight**
It would be beneficial to your health to lose some weight.

■ **Fat**
It's really important to lose weight since your health may suffer at your current weight.

■ **Very Fat**
Being this overweight could be a serious risk to your health. You urgently need to lose weight and would do well to see your doctor or a dietitian.

© Health Education Authority 1994, reproduced by permission.

Figure 10.2. *Height/Weight Chart*

158

reevaluate these changes again. In the meantime, accept that this is the right decision for you at this time, and focus your attention on other goals.

If you decide that now *is* the right time, start by changing those things that feel most *comfortable to you.* You don't have to do it all right away. Remember, slow and steady wins the race.

To help get started, keep track of what you are currently doing. For example, write down your daily routine to identify where you might be able to add some exercise. Or keep a food diary for a week to see what, when, why, and how much you eat. This can help you identify how and where to make changes in your eating habits, as well as how to shop for and prepare meals. The diary may also help you look at the relationship between your eating patterns and emotions or other symptoms. The sample food–mood diary on page 161 may be useful. Next, choose only one or two things to change first. Allow yourself time to get used to these and then add more changes. The goal setting and action planning skills discussed in Chapter 1 will help with this.

Common Problems with Eating for Health

"I enjoy eating out (or I hate to cook), so how do I know if I'm eating well?"

Whether it's because you don't have time, you hate to cook, or you just don't have the energy to go grocery shopping and prepare meals, eating out may suit your needs. This is not necessarily bad if you know which choices are healthy ones.

Here are tips on eating out:

- Select restaurants that offer variety and flexibility in types of food and methods of preparation. Feel free to ask what is in a dish and how it is prepared, especially if you are eating in a restaurant where the dishes are new or different from what you are used to.

- Plan what type of food you will eat and how much. (You can bring the left-overs home.)

- Choose items low in fat, sodium, and sugar or ask if they can be prepared that way. For example, appetisers might include steamed seafood or raw vegetables without fancy sauces or dips, or bread without butter. You may request salad with dressing on the side, or bring your own oil-free dressing. For an entrée, you might try broiled, barbecued, baked, grilled, or steamed dishes. Choose fish or poultry over red meat. Avoid breaded, fried, sautéed, or creamy dishes. Choose dishes whose ingredients are listed. Instead of a whole dinner, consider ordering à la carte and lots of vegetables (without butter or sauces). For dessert, select fruit or non-fat yogurt. You might split an entrée or a dessert with someone else.

- Order first so that you aren't tempted to change your order after hearing what others have selected.

- If you want fast food, choose salads with dressing on the side, baked potatoes instead of fries, juice or milk instead of soda, and frozen yogurt instead of ice cream.

"I snack while I watch TV (or read)."

If you know this is a problem for you, plan ahead by preparing healthier snacks. For example, rather than eating "junk" food like crisps and cookies, munch on fresh fruit, raw vegetables, or air-popped popcorn. Try designating specific areas at home and work as "eating areas" and limit your eating to those areas.

159

"I eat when I'm bored/depressed/feeling lonely, etc."

Many people find comfort in food. Some people eat when they don't have anything else to do or just to fill in time. Some eat when they're feeling down or upset. Unfortunately, at these times, you often lose track of what and how much you eat. These are also the times when celery sticks, apples, or popcorn never seem to do the trick. Instead, you start out with a full bag of potato crisps and, by the end of an hour, have only crumbs left. To help control these urges, try to:

160

- Keep a food-mood diary. Every day, list what, how much, and when you eat. Note how you are feeling when you have the urge to eat. Try to spot patterns so you can anticipate when you will want to eat without really being hungry. (The sample diary on page 161 can be used for this.)
- Make a plan for when these situations arise. If you catch yourself feeling bored, go for a short walk, work on a jigsaw puzzle, or otherwise occupy your mind and hands. This may be a time to practise a distraction technique.

"Healthy food doesn't taste the same as real food. The healthy stuff just doesn't fill me up!"

Just because you are trying to make healthier food choices does not mean that you will never again eat your favourite foods. Follow the Balance of Good Health and eat in moderation. Healthier eating only means that you will change some of the ways you prepare these foods, as well as what you buy at the supermarket. Additional information is available in the references at the end of this chapter.

"But I LOVE to cook!"

If you love to cook, you are in luck. This is your opportunity to take a new cooking class or to buy a new recipe book on healthy cooking. Again, experiment with different ways to modify your favourite recipes, increasing the amount of fruit and vegetables you use and limiting the amount of fat, sugar and salt.

"I'm living alone now, and I'm not used to cooking for one. I find myself over-eating so food isn't wasted."

This can be a problem, especially if you are not use to measuring ingredients. You may be overeating or eating a "second dinner" to fill time. Or maybe you are one of those people who will eat for as long as the food is in front of you. Whatever the reason, here are some ways to help you to deal with the extra food:

Food–Mood Diary

Date	Time	What I Ate	Where I Ate	Mood/Feelings

161

Things That Will Enable Me to Make the Desired Changes	Things That Will Make It Difficult for Me to Change
Example: I have the support of family and friends.	*Example:* The holidays are coming up and there are too many gatherings to prepare for.

162

- Don't put the serving dishes on the table. Take as much as you feel you can comfortably eat and bring only your plate to the table.

- As soon as you've finished eating, wrap up what you haven't eaten and put it in the refrigerator or freezer. This way, you have leftovers for the next day or whenever you don't want to cook.

- Invite friends over for dinner once in a while so that you can share food and each other's company, or plan a potluck supper with neighbours or relatives.

- Attend your community or church meals.

163

Common Problems with Losing Weight

"I wish I could lose ten pounds in the next two weeks. I want to look good for . . . ."

Sound familiar? Almost everyone who has tried to lose weight wants to lose it quickly. This is a hard pattern to break because, although it may be possible to lose 5 to 10 pounds (2–5 kg) in one or two weeks, it is not healthy nor is it likely to stay off. Rapid weight loss is usually water loss, which can be dangerous, causing the body to become dehydrated. When this happens you may also experience other symptoms such as light-headedness, headaches, fatigue, and poor sleep. Rather than doing this to yourself, try a different approach—one employing realistic goal-setting and positive self-talk. (These are discussed in greater detail in Chapters 1 and 3, respectively.) Here are some approaches to sensible weight loss:

- Set your goal to lose weight *gradually,* just one or two pounds (1 kg) a week.

- Identify the specific steps you will take to lose this weight, for example, increasing activities and/or changing what you eat.

- Change your self-talk from "I really need to lose 10 pounds right away" to "Losing this weight gradually will help me keep it off for good."

- Be patient. You didn't gain weight overnight, so you can't expect to lose it overnight.

"I can lose the first several pounds relatively painlessly, but I just can't seem to lose those last few pounds."

This can be frustrating and puzzling, especially when you have been eating healthy and staying active. However, it is quite common and usually means that your body has adapted to your new calorie intake and activity level. While your first impulse may be to cut your calorie intake even further, it probably won't help and could be unhealthy. Remember, you want to make changes you can live with.

Ask yourself how much of a difference one, two, or even five pounds will really make. If you are feeling good, the chances are you don't need to lose more weight. It is not unhealthy to live with a few extra pounds, if you are staying active and eating low-fat foods. You may already be at a healthy weight given your body size and shape. Also, you may be replacing fat with muscle, which weighs more. However, if you decide that these pounds must go, try the following:

- Modify your goal so that you maintain your weight for a few weeks; try to lose a pound more gradually over the next few weeks.

- Try adding to your physical activity exercise goals, especially if the current activity you do has become easy. Increasing your activity level will help you to use more calories and maintain your muscle mass. Less weight will be stored in the form of fat. (Tips for safely increasing your exercise are found in Chapter 6.)

- Again, be patient and allow your body time to adjust to your new patterns.

- Watch your portion sizes and eat a low fat diet based on plenty of fruit, vegetables and starchy foods. See page 143 about the Balance of Good Health.

"I always feel so deprived of the foods I love when I try to lose weight."

The key to reaching and maintaining a healthy weight is to make changes you can tolerate, even enjoy. This means they must suit your lifestyle and needs. Unfortunately, when thinking about losing weight, most of us tend to think of all the things we *can't* eat. Change this way of thinking now! There are probably as many (if not more) enjoyable foods you CAN eat than ones you should limit. Sometimes it is just a matter of learning to prepare foods differently, rather than eliminating them completely. If you like to cook, this is your opportunity to become creative, learning new recipes or finding ways to change old ones. There are many good cookbooks on the market today to help you make this process more enjoyable. Some of these tips were outlined earlier in this chapter, and more can be found in the references listed at the end of the chapter.

"I eat too fast or I finish eating before everyone and find myself reaching for seconds."

Eating too fast happens for a couple of reasons. One may be that you are limiting yourself to only two or three meals a day, not eating or drinking between meals. This can leave you so hungry at mealtime that you practically inhale your food. Another reason may be that you have not had a chance to slow down and relax before eating. Slowing down your eating can help you decrease the amount of food you eat. If you find you are too hungry, feeling stressed out, or in a hurry, try one or more of the following:

- Try not to skip meals. In this way you are less likely to overeat at the next meal.

- Allow yourself to snack on healthier choices between meals. In fact, plan your snacks for mid morning or afternoon. Fruit or raw vegetables (e.g. carrot sticks) make a good snack.

- Eat more frequent, smaller meals. This may also be easier on your digestive system, which won't be overwhelmed by a large meal eaten in a hurry.

- Chew your food well. Food is an enjoyable necessity! Chewing your food well also eases the burden on your digestive system.

- Drink plenty of water! Six to eight glasses of water per day is recommended. This helps you to eat less and helps prevent medication side-effects, aids elimination, and keeps the kidneys functioning properly.

- Try a relaxation method about a half hour before you eat. Several methods are discussed in Chapter 3.

Common Problems with Gaining Weight

"I don't know how to add pounds."

Here are some ways to increase the amount of calories and/or nutrients you eat. These may also add some fat to your eating plan. Check with your doctor or a nutritionist to see which of the following tips are appropriate for you.

- Eat smaller meals more often during the day.
- Don't skip meals.
- Eat high-calorie foods first at each meal, saving the vegetables, fruits, and beverages for later.

- Snack on calorie-rich foods such as avocados, nuts, seeds, nut butter, or dried fruits.
- Drink high-calorie beverages such as milk shakes, malt drinks, and fruit whips.
- Eat high-protein foods, such as meat, fish, nuts or dairy products.
- Use milk to prepare creamed dishes with meat, fish, or poultry.
- Add meat, fish, cheese or nuts to salads.
- Add milk or milk powder to sauces, gravies, cereals, soups, and casseroles.
- Use melted cheese on vegetables and other dishes.
- Add butter, margarine, oils, and creams to dishes (1–3 tablespoons [15–45 ml] per day).
- Use protein, vitamin, and mineral supplements if needed (consult with your doctor or a nutritionist).
- Eating something is better than nothing at all — try to think of something you really enjoy and would find tasty.

"Food doesn't taste as good as before."

If you have had a tracheostomy, are receiving oxygen through a nasal cannula, or are taking certain medicines, you may have noticed a decrease in your taste sensations. To compensate, you may have also noticed that you've been increasing the amount of salt you add to your foods. To avoid this, try enhancing the flavours of foods by

- Experimenting with herbs, spices, and other seasonings. Start with just about ¼ teaspoon (5ml) in a dish for four people.
- Modifying recipes to include a wide variety of ingredients to make the food look and taste more appealing.
- Chewing your food well. This will allow the food to remain in your mouth longer and provide more stimulation to your taste buds.

If the decline in taste is keeping you from getting essential nutrients, you may need to adjust the calorie content of these foods. Tips for doing this are mentioned above.

"It takes so long to prepare meals. By the time I'm done, I'm too tired to eat."

If this is a problem for you, then it's time to develop a plan, because you need to eat to maintain your energy level. Here are some hints to help:

166

- Plan your meals for the week.

- Then go to the grocery store and buy everything you will need.

- Break your food preparation into steps, resting in between.

- Cook enough for two, three, or even more servings, especially if it's something you really like.

- Freeze the extra portions in single-serving sizes. On the days when you are really tired, thaw and reheat one of these pre-cooked, frozen meals.

- Ask for help, especially for those big meals or at family gatherings.

167

"Sometimes eating causes discomfort." Or, "I'm afraid I'll become short of breath while I'm eating."

People who experience shortness of breath or who find it difficult and physically uncomfortable to eat meals tend to eat less and may be underweight. For some, eating a large meal causes indigestion. Indigestion, along with a full stomach, reduces the space your breathing muscles have to expand and contract. This can aggravate breathing problems. If this is a problem for you:

- Try eating four to six smaller meals a day, rather than the usual three larger meals. This reduces the amount of oxygen you need to chew and digest each meal.

- Avoid foods that produce wind or make you feel bloated. You can determine which foods affect you this way by trying different foods and observing the results. Often these foods include vegetables such as cabbage, broccoli, brussels sprouts, varieties of onions, beans, and fruits like raw apples, melons, and avocados, especially if eaten in large quantities.

- Eat slowly, taking small bites and chewing your food well. You should also pause occasionally during a meal. Eating quickly to avoid an episode of shortness of breath can actually bring one on. Slowing down and breathing evenly reduces the amount of air you swallow while eating.

- Practise a relaxation exercise about half an hour before mealtime, or take time out for a few deep breaths during the meal.

"I can't eat much in one sitting."

There is no real need to eat only three meals a day. In fact, for many it is recommended that you eat four to six smaller meals. If you choose to do this, include "no fuss", high-calorie snacks like milk, bread, and fruits or liquid protein shakes as part of these extra meals. If you still can't finish a whole meal, be sure to eat the portion of your meal that is highest in calories first. Save the vegetables, fruits, and beverages for last.

Common Problems with Maintaining Your Weight

168

"I've been on a LOT of diets before and lost a lot of weight. But I've always gained it back, and then some. It's so frustrating, and I just don't understand WHY this happens!!!"

Many of you have probably experienced this problem, which occurs because the diet was short-term and calorie-restricted; it did not emphasise changes in eating habits. In fact, this is the problem with many "diets". They involve drastic changes in both what is eaten and the way it is eaten that they cannot be tolerated for long. Because your body does not know when more food will be available again, it reacts physiologically to this deprivation, slowing its metabolism to adapt to a smaller amount of food energy. Then, when you've had enough of the diet, or have lost the weight and return to your old eating habits, you gain the weight back. Sometimes you even gain back more weight than you lost. Again, the body is responding physiologically, replenishing its stores, usually in the form of fat. This fat serves as a concentrated energy source to be called upon again when calories are restricted. This causes the weight to go up and down in cycles which, as mentioned before, is unhealthy and very discouraging.

This situation is further complicated by feelings of deprivation, as you probably had to give up your favourite foods. Therefore, when you reach your goal weight, you begin to eat all of those foods again freely and most likely in larger quantities.

The key to maintaining a healthy weight is developing healthy eating habits that are enjoyable to you and fit into your lifestyle. We have already discussed many of these tips earlier in this chapter. Here are a few more:

- Set a small weight-range goal that you consider to be healthy for *you*. Weights fluctuate naturally. By setting a range, you will allow yourself some flexibility.

- Monitor your activity level. Once you have lost some weight, exercise three to five times a week to improve your chances of keeping the weight off. If possible, gradually increase your activity level.

- Watch your portion size and make sure you are following a low fat diet based on plenty of fruits and vegetables. See page 143 about the Balance of Good Health.

"I do okay maintaining my weight for a short time. Then something happens beyond my control, and my concerns about what I eat become insignificant. Before I know it I've slipped back into my old eating habits."

If you had only a little slip, don't worry about it. Just continue as if nothing happened. If the slip is longer, try to evaluate why: is there a situation or circumstance requiring a lot of attention now? If so, weight management may be taking a back seat for a while. This is not a problem. The sooner you realise this the better, and try to set a date when you will start your weight management programme again. You may even want to join a support group and stay with it for at least four to six months. If so, look for one that:

- Emphasises good nutrition and the use of a wide variety of foods
- Emphasises changes in eating habits and patterns
- Gives support in the form of ongoing meetings or long-term follow-up

Eating well does not mean that you are forever forbidden to eat certain foods. It means learning to eat a variety of foods in the right quantities to maintain your health and/or better manage your disease symptoms. The Balance of Good Health emphasises eating a wide variety of foods in moderation. For many people, a healthier diet will mean eating more fruit and vegetables and reducing the amount of fat, sugar and salt they eat. These changes are also important for effective weight management. If you choose to make some of the changes suggested in this chapter, remember that you should not feel like you are punishing yourself, nor that this is a life sentence to boring, bland food. As a self-manager, it's up to you to find the changes that are best for you. And if you experience setbacks, identify the problems and work at resolving them. Remember, if you *really* want to, you *can* do it!

Resources

There is so much information available commercially and on the world wide web on diets and healthy eating that it is sometimes difficult to know what to believe. The website, www.quackwatch.com is useful to check claims made about food supplements. Other resources include:

- The Food Standards Agency has various leaflets on food related issues. See http://www.foodstandards.gov.uk

- NHS Direct online www.nhsdirect.nhs.uk has a great deal of information on healthy eating, diet and nutrition

169

- The press generally keeps a watchful eye on diet and health issues. The BBC website is a good way to keep up with health in the news, www.bbc.co.uk/health/nutrition

- Most GP surgeries and health centres have information on general diets and special diets for people with certain conditions

- The disease-specific supplements to the handbook provide details on dietary issues related to different diseases; ask your Expert Patients Programme Trainers for these booklets

• • •

Suggested Further Reading

General

British Heart Foundation. *The Light-Hearted Cookbook* and *The Everyday Light-Hearted Cookbook*. London: British Heart Foundation. Write to BHF, 14 Fitzharding Street, London W1H 6DH. Tel: 010 7935 0185

British Heart Foundation. "So you want to lose weight . . . for good." British Heart Foundation, 14 Fitzardinge Street, LondonW1H 6DH. Tel 0207 935 0185.

Brody, Jane. *Jane Brody's Nutrition Book*. New York: Bantam, 1982.

Deutsch, Ronald M., and Judi S. Morrill, Ph. D. *Realities of Nutrition*. Rev. ed. Palo Alto, Calif.: Bull Publishing, 1993.

Escott-Stump, Sylvia. *Nutrition and Diagnosis-Related Care*. Lippincott Williams and Wilkins, 1997.

Hodgkin, John E. (Editor), et al. *Pulmonary Rehabilitation*. Lippincott Williams and Wilkins.

Peters, James A., Kenneth Burke, and Debra White. "Nutrition and the pulmonary patient." In *Pulmonary Rehabilitation: Guidelines to Success*, edited by John E. Hodgkin, Eileen G. Zorn, and Gerilynn L. Conners. Stoneham, Mass.: Butterworth Publishers, 1984.

Williams, Sue R. S. *Essentials of Nutrition and Diet Therapy*. St. Louis, Mo.: Times Mirror/Mosby College Publishing, 1990.

Vegetarian Eating

Lappé, Frances. *Diet for a Small Planet*. New York: Ballantine, 1985.

Robertson, Laurel, Carol Flinders, and Bronwen Godfrey. *Laurel's Kitchen: A Handbook for Vegetarian Cookery and Nutrition*. New York: Bantam, 1978.

Weight Control

Ferguson, James M. *Habits Not Diets*. 2nd ed. Palo Alto, Calif.: Bull Publishing, 1988.

Nash, Joyce D, *The New Maximize Your Body Potential*. 2nd ed. Palo Alto, Calif.: Bull Publishing, 1997.

Nelson, Miriam E. *Strong Women Stay Slim*. New York: Bantam Books,1998.

CHAPTER
11

Managing Your Medicines

A N IMPLICATION OF HAVING A CHRONIC ILLNESS is usually having one or more medicines prescribed. Thus a very important management task is to understand your medicines and to use them appropriately. This chapter will help you do just that.

A Few General Words About Medicines

Although advertising prescription medicines direct to the public is not legal in the UK there is a great deal of advertising of non-prescription or as they are often know "over-the-counter" (OTC) medicines. For example ibuprofen is being promoted in a number of different smart packages with claims for its pain relieving properties. There is also a huge public interest in the development and availability of prescription only medicines. This is reflected in the number of column inches devoted to discussing Viagra (for impotence), the so-called COX-2s (for arthritis), statins (for cardiovascular disease) and β-interferon (for MS). As if this was not sufficiently confusing, it is only recently that the term "medicine" has been reserved to describe chemicals taken as a therapy, and the term "drug" reserved for chemicals taken without medical supervision or illegally. In addition, we have all heard the messages about avoiding overdoses and excess medicines. Steering a path through this is not easy.

Your body is its own healer and, if given time to work, most common symptoms and disorders will improve. The prescriptions filled by the body's internal pharmacy are frequently the safest and most effective treatment. So patience, careful self-observation and monitoring can be excellent therapeutic choices for you and your prescriber to take.

It is also true that medicines can be a very important part of managing a chronic illness. These medicines do not cure the disease. They generally have one or more of the following purposes.

1. *They help symptoms through their chemical actions.* For example, a bronchodilator inhaler delivers medicines that expand the airways and make it easier to breathe, or a GTN tablet expands the blood vessels allowing more blood to reach the heart, quieting angina.

2. Other medicines are aimed at *preventing further problems.* For example, medicines that thin the blood help prevent blood clots, which can cause strokes and heart problems.

3. A third type of medicine *helps to improve symptoms or slow the disease process.* For example, non-steroidal anti-inflammatory medicines (NSAIDs) can help arthritis by quieting the inflammatory process. Likewise, digitalis can help regulate and strengthen the heart beat.

4. Finally, there are medicines to *provide substances that the body is no longer producing adequately.* This is how insulin is used by someone with diabetes.

In all cases, the purpose of the medicine is to lessen the consequences of disease *or* to slow its course or to prevent it occuring. You may not be aware that the medicines are doing anything. For example, if a medicine is slowing the course of the disease, you may not feel anything, and this may lead you to believe that the medicine isn't doing anything (for example medicines to treat high blood pressure). It is important to continue taking your medicines, even if you cannot see how they are helping. If this concerns you, ask your doctor or pharmacist.

We pay a price for having such powerful tools. Besides being helpful, all medicines have some undesirable side effects. Some are predictable and minor, and some are unexpected and life-threatening. From 5% to 10% of all hospital admissions are due to the side effects of medicines or medicine reactions.

What Is a Side Effect?

A side effect is *any* effect other than the one you want. Usually, it is an undesirable effect. Examples of side effects are stomach problems, constipation or diarrhoea, sleepiness or dizziness. It is important to know the common side effects for the medicines you take. Sometimes people say they can't or won't take a medicine because of possible side effects. This is a reasonable response. However, before making a decision to stop a medicine or refusing to take it, there are some questions you should ask yourself and your doctor.

Are the benefits from this medicine more important than the side effects?

The use of chemotherapy for people with cancer is a good example. While these medicines have side effects, many people still choose the medicines because of their life-saving qualities. To take or not to take a medicine is your decision. However, it should always be looked upon as "will I be better off with the medicine despite its side effects?"

Are there some ways of avoiding the side effects or making them less severe?

Many times the way you take the medicine, for example, with food or without food, can make a difference. Ask your doctor or pharmacist for advice on this question.

Are there other medicines with the same benefits but fewer side effects?

Often there are several medicines that do the same thing but react differently in different people. Unfortunately, no one knows how a medicine will react in you until you have taken it. Therefore, your doctor may have to try several medicines before hitting on the one that is best for you. For this reason, when getting a new medicine, it is good practise to try out a prescription for only a week or two before moving to a month's supply. In this way, if the medicine does not work out, you will not have wasted time or money.

Taking Multiple Medicines

It is not uncommon for patients with multiple problems to be taking multiple medicaines: a medicine to lower blood pressure, anti-inflammatory medicines for arthritis, a pill for angina, a bronchodilator for asthma, antacids for heartburn, a tranquilizer for anxiety, plus a handful of over-the-counter remedies and herbs. *Remember, the more medicines you are taking, the greater the risk of side effects.* Fortunately, it is often possible to reduce the number of medicines and the associated risks. It requires forging effective partnerships with your doctor and community pharmacist. This involves participation in determining the need for the medicine, selecting the medicine, properly using the medicine, and reporting back to your doctor and the pharmacist the effect of the medicine.

173

One of the roles of the community pharmacist is improving the health of and protecting the public. They are expert at checking for medicine interactions and frequently advise the GPs. Increasingly pharmacists are making themselves available to discuss the concerns of their patients.

An individual's response to a particular medicine varies depending on age, metabolism, activity level, other medicines that are being taken, and the waxing and waning of symptoms characteristic of most chronic diseases. Many medicines are prescribed on an as-needed ("PRN") basis so that you need to know when to begin and end treatment and how much medicine to take. You need to work out a plan with your doctor/pharmacist to suit your individual needs.

For most medicines, *your doctor/pharmacist depends on you* to report what effect, if any, the medicine has on your symptoms and what side effects you may be experiencing. Based on that critical information your medicines may be continued, increased, discontinued, or otherwise changed. In a good doctor–patient partnership, there is a continuing flow of information. There are important things you need to let your doctor know and critical information you need to receive.

Unfortunately, this vital interchange is too often shortchanged. Studies indicate that fewer than 5% of patients receiving new prescriptions asked any questions of their doctors or pharmacists. Doctors tend to interpret patient silence as understanding and satisfaction with the information received. Mishaps often occur because patients do not receive adequate information about their medicines and don't understand how to take them properly or fail to follow instructions given to them. Safe, effective medicine use depends on your understanding of the proper use, the risks, and the necessary precautions associated with each medicine you take. *You must ask questions.*

Many patients are reluctant to ask their doctor questions, fearing to appear ignorant or to be challenging the doctor's authority. But asking questions is a necessary part of a healthy doctor–patient relationship.

The goal of treatment is to maximize the benefit and minimize the risks. This means taking the fewest medicines, in the lowest effective doses, for the shortest period of time. Whether the medicines you take are helpful or harmful often depends on how much you know about your medicines and how well you communicate with your doctor.

What You Need to TELL Your Doctor

Even if your doctor doesn't ask, there is certain vital information you should mention to her or him.

174

Are you taking any medicines?

Report to your doctor and dentist *all* the prescription and non-prescription medicines you are taking, including birth control pills, vitamins, aspirin, antacids, laxatives, and herbal remedies. This is especially important if you are seeing more than one prescriber. Each one may not know what the others have prescribed. Knowing all the medicines and herbs you are taking is essential to correct diagnosis and treatment. For example, if you have symptoms like nausea or diarrhoea, sleeplessness or drowsiness, dizziness or memory loss, impotence or fatigue, they may be due to a side effect of a medicine rather than a disease. It is critical for your doctor to know what medicines you are taking to help avoid problems from medicine interactions. It is helpful to carry an up-to-date list of all the medicines you are taking. Saying that you are taking "the little green pills" usually doesn't help identify the medicine. Sometimes it is beneficial to bring in all your medicines (including over-the-counter medicines) in a bag so that your doctor can review them, advising you which to continue and which to stop or discard. If you write a list of all the medicines you are taking and their dosages, your doctor doesn't have to spend valuable minutes looking through your medical notes. The list should include any medicines prescribed in hospital. When the list is up to date it should also be shown to the pharmacist. [Note: If you have medicines to discard take them to the chemist for safe disposal.]

Have you had allergic or unusual reactions to any medicines?

Describe any symptoms or unusual reactions you have had to any medicines taken in the past. Be specific: which medicine and exactly what type of reaction. A rash, fever, or wheezing that develops after taking a medicine is often a true allergic reaction. The severity of allergic reactions can vary considerably. If any of these develop, call your doctor at once. On the other hand, nausea, ringing in the ears, light-headedness and agitation, are more likely to be side effects rather than true allergies to a medicine.

Do you have any major chronic diseases or other medical conditions?

Many diseases can interfere with the action of a medicine or increase the risk of using certain medicines. Diseases involving the kidneys or liver are especially important to mention since these diseases can slow the metabolism of many medicines and increase toxic effects. Your doctor may also avoid certain medicines if you now or in the past have had such diseases as hypertension, peptic ulcer, asthma, heart disease, diabetes, or prostate problems. Also be sure to let your doctor know if you might be pregnant or are breast-feeding since many medicines cannot be safely used in those situations.

What medicines were tried in the past to treat your disease?

If you have a chronic disease, it is a good idea to keep your own written record of what medicines were tried in the past to help manage the condition and what the effects were. Knowing your past responses to various medicines will help guide the doctor's recommendation of any new medicines. However, just because a medicine did not work successfully in the past does not necessarily mean that it can't be tried again. Diseases change and may become more responsive to treatment.

What You Need to ASK Your Doctor

Do I really need this medicine?

Some doctors decide to prescribe medicines not because they are really necessary, but because they think this is what patients want and expect. Doctors often feel pressure to do something for the patient, so they reach for the prescription pad. Don't pressure your doctor for medicines. If your doctor doesn't prescribe a medicine, consider that good news rather than a sign of rejection or disinterest. Ask about herbs and other nonmedicine alternatives. Many conditions can be treated in a variety of ways, and your doctor can explain alternative choices. In some cases lifestyle changes such as exercise, diet and stress management should be considered before making a decision. When any treatment is recommended, also ask what the likely consequences are if you postpone treatment. Sometimes the best medicine is none at all.

What is the name of the medicine?

If a medicine is prescribed, it is important that you know its name. Write down both the brand name and the generic (or chemical) name. If the medicine you get from the pharmacy doesn't have the same name(s) as the one your doctor prescribed, ask the pharmacist to explain the difference.

What is the medicine supposed to do?

Your doctor should tell you why the medicine is being prescribed and how it might be expected to help you. Is the medicine intended to prolong your life, completely or partially relieve your symptoms, or improve your ability to function? For example, if you are given a diuretic for high blood pressure, the medicine is given primarily to prevent later complications (i.e. stroke or heart disease) rather than to stop your headache. On the other hand, if you are given paracetamol, the purpose is to help ease pain. You should also know how soon you should expect results from the medicine. Some medicines which treat infections or inflammation may take several days to a week to show improvement, while antidepressant medicines and some arthritis medicines typically take several weeks to begin working. On the other hand some medicines start to have a noticeable effect immediately.

How and when do I take the medicine and for how long?

Understanding how much of the medicine to take and how often to take it is critical to the safe, effective use of medicines. Does "every six hours" mean "every six hours while awake"? Should the medicine be taken before meals, with meals, or between meals? What should you do if you accidentally miss a dose? Should you skip it, take a double dose next time, or take it as soon as you remember? Should you continue taking the medicine until the symptoms subside or until the medicine is finished?

The answers to such questions are very important. For example, if you are taking a non-steroidal anti-inflammatory medicine for arthritis, you may feel better within a few days, but should still take the medicine as prescribed to maintain the anti-inflammatory effect. Or, if you abruptly stop taking steroid medicines used for severe asthma as soon as the wheezing improves, you are likely to relapse. If you are using an inhaled medicine for treatment of asthma, the way you use the inhaler critically determines how much of the medicine actually gets into your lungs. Taking the medicine properly is vital. Yet when patients were surveyed in the USA, nearly 40% reported that they were not told by their doctors how to take the medicine or how much to take. If you are not sure about your prescription, talk to your doctor or community pharmacist. Such discussions are never considered a bother.

What foods, drinks, other medicines, or activities should I avoid while taking this medicine?

The presence of food in the stomach may help protect the stomach from some medicines while it may render other medicines ineffective. For example, milk products or antacids block the absorption of the antibiotic tetracycline, so this medicine is best taken on an empty stomach. Some medicines may make you more sensitive to the sun, putting you at increased risk for sunburn. Ask whether the medicine prescribed will interfere with driving safely. Other medicines you may be taking, even over-the-counter medicines and alcohol, can either amplify or inhibit the effects of the prescribed medicine. Taking aspirin along with an anti-coagulant medicine can result in enhanced blood-thinning and possible bleeding. The more medicines you are taking, the greater the chance of an undesirable medicine interaction. So talk to your pharmacist about possible medicine-medicine and medicine-food interactions.

What are the most common side effects, and what should I do if they occur?

All medicines have side effects. You need to know what symptoms to be on the lookout for and what action to take if they develop. Should you seek immediate medical care, discontinue the medicine, continue to take the medicine or call your doctor? While the doctor cannot be expected to tell you every possible adverse reaction, the more common and important ones should be discussed. Unfortunately, a recent survey in the USA showed that 70% of patients starting a new medicine did not recall being told by their doctors or pharmacists about precautions and possible side effects. So it may be up to you to ask.

Are there any tests necessary to monitor the use of this medicine?

Most medicines are monitored by the improvement or worsening of symptoms. However, some medicines can disrupt body chemistry before any telltale symptoms develop. Sometimes these adverse reactions have to be detected by laboratory tests such as blood counts or liver function tests. In addition, the levels of some medicines in the blood need to be measured periodically to make sure you are getting the right amounts. Ask your doctor if the medicine being prescribed has any of these special requirements.

Can an alternative or generic medicine that is less expensive be prescribed?

Every medicine has at least two names, a generic name and a brand name. The generic name is the name used to refer to the medicine in the scientific literature. The brand name is the company's unique name for the medicine. When a medicine company develops a new medicine, it is granted exclusive rights to produce that medicine for 17 years. In this time they will recover the costs of developing the medicine. After this 17-year period has expired, other companies may market chemical equivalents of that medicine. These generic medicines are generally considered as safe and effective as the original brand-name medicine, but often cost half as much or less. GPs and consultants are encouraged to use generics as much as possible to keep the expenditure on medicines as low as possible. Sometimes it is cheaper for you to buy the appropriate medicine as an OTC (over-the-counter) rather than paying the prescription charge. This does not mean it is a lesser medicine. The guidance on how and when to take it should be followed as closely as before.

Is there any written information about the medicine?

Realistically, your doctor may not have time to answer all of your questions in great detail. Even if your doctor carefully answers the questions, it is difficult for anyone to remember all of this information.

All medicines come with a patient information leaflet. Some of these are excellent and will also give you an advice line to call for further information. Some leaflets are very legalistic and list every side effect that has ever happened to anyone, anywhere. These can create unnecessary anxiety. Usually, the pharmacists are the best source of information about medicines. Increasingly they have data on their computers that they will print off to supply you with additional information about your medicines. There are also useful websites, for example www.femail.co.uk and www.medicine-chest.co.uk that you can go to for information. However, information is more than the words and even when you know a lot about a medicine it is worth getting the pharmacist's opinion.

In some cases where specialist nurses are involved, as in diabetes and multiple sclerosis, they are available by phone for advice about your medicines. There are many sources of information and advice available. Some useful books are listed at the end of the chapter, but don't overlook voluntary organisations' helplines. They usually have leaflets and guidance written specially for people like you.

Pharmacists Are An Underutilised Resource

Pharmacists are the health care specialists on medicines, how they act in your body, and how they interact with each other. Their roles are likely to grow in coming years. Pharmacists you can talk to fall into two categories, hospital and community. It is okay to talk to the hospital pharmacist about your medicines. This is not often done but many value direct contact with patients and are a mine of information. Community pharmacists (dispensing chemists as they used to be called) are increasingly understanding this role to be part of their service. It is smart to find a pharmacist whose services you like and to stay with them. Gradually they will build up a picture of your medicine requirements and be in a good position to advise you when asked. As a self-manager, don't forget the pharmacists. They are helpful consultants.

Prescriptions and Prescription Charges

NHS prescriptions carry a £6.10 charge per item dispensed by the community pharmacist. The number of items can mean that the monthly medicine bill is considerable. There are number of ways to keep these costs to a minimum.

The first is to check that you have to pay at all. There are several exemptions. You are automatically exempt if you are

- under 16 or under 19 and in fulltime education
- 60 or over
- getting income support or income based Job Seekers Allowance
- getting a maximum award of working families tax credit, or a disabled person's tax credit or the amount taken off the maximum is £71 per week or less
- the partner (or dependent child) of someone who gets one of the benefits in the above list
- you are an asyulum seeker getting government support, or their partner or dependent child

You also qualify for an exemption certificate if you are:

- an expectant mother
- a woman who had a child in the last year
- someone with a specified condition or are housebound with a continuing disability
- a war/service pensioner needing treatment of accepted disabilities
- or qualify under the low income scheme

Specified conditions are:

- a permanent physical disability that prevents you from leaving your home except with the help of someone else
- fistulas or stomas that require dressings or an appliance
- diabetes when the control is not by diet alone
- conditions where supplemental thyroid hormone is necessary
- epilepsy requiring continuous anti-convulsive therapy
- hyperthyroidism, hypopituitism, myasthenia gravis and hypoadrenalism

The forms needed to claim these exemptions come from the pharmacist. The pharmacist is required to ask you for evidence that you qualify for an exemption.

Other than these exemptions the only way of actually reducing your prescription charges is to buy a prepayment certificate. These cover all your prescription costs for the relevant period. A four month prepayment certificates costs £31.90 and a year certificate costs £87.60. These certificates save you money if you need more than 14 items a year or more than 5 in four months. There is just one snag. There is a ceiling on the income you can have and be entitled to these certificates. However the calculation is complex and does not apply to most people.

A word of warning. Prescription forms are now being audited and false declarations followed up. Be careful to read the exemptions on the form carefully. If you have questions about your entitlement, ask the pharmacist.

Finally, the complexities of benefits and exemptions are an example of what needs to be considered when a full welfare benefits entitlement is calculated. If this is done thoroughly, there are considerable financial gains possible.

Remembering to Take Your Medicine

No matter what medicine is prescribed, it won't do you any good if you don't take it. Nearly half of all medicines are not taken regularly as prescribed. There are many reasons why this occurs: forgetfulness, lack of clear instructions, complicated dosing schedules, bothersome side effects, prescription charges, beliefs about medicines, and so on. Whatever the reason, if you are having trouble or worries taking your medicines as prescribed, discuss this with your doctor/pharmacist. Often, simple adjustments can make it easier. For example, if you are taking five different medicines, sometimes one or more can be eliminated. If you are taking one medicine three times a day and another four times a day, your doctor may be able to simplify the regimen. Understanding more about your medicines, including how they can help you, may also help motivate you to take them regularly.

If forgetting to take your medicines is a major problem, then here are some suggestions:

- *Place a post-it reminder* next to your toothbrush, on the meal table, in your lunch box, or in some other place where you're likely to "stumble over" it. Or you might put a reminder note on the bathroom mirror, the refrigerator door, the coffee maker, the television, or some other conspicuous place. If you link taking the medicine with some well-established habit such as meal times or watching your favourite television programme, you'll be more likely to remember.

- *Make a medicine chart* containing each medicine you are taking and when you take it. You can then tick off each medicine as you take it noting the time and date. You might also *buy a "medicines organiser"* at the pharmacy. This container separates pills according to the time of day they should be taken. You then fill the organiser once a week so that all of your pills are ready to take at the proper time. A quick glance at the organiser lets you know if you have missed any doses and prevents double dosing.

- *Get a watch that can be set to beep at pill-taking time.* There are also "high-tech" medicine containers available that beep at a pre-programmed time to remind you to take your medicine.

- *Ask other family or household members to help remind you* to take your medicines.

- *Don't run out* of your medicines. When you get a new prescription, mark on your calendar the date a week before your medicines will run out. This will serve as a reminder to get your next refill. Don't wait until the last pill.

If you plan to travel, *put a note in your luggage reminding you* to pack your pills. Also, *take along an extra prescription* in your carry-on luggage in case you lose your pills or your luggage.

Self-Medication

In addition to medicines prescribed by your doctor, you, like most people, may take nonprescription or over-the-counter (OTC) medicines and herbal remedies. In fact, within every two-week period in the USA nearly 70% of people will self-medicate with one or more medicines. Many OTC medicines are highly effective and may even be recommended by your doctor. But if you self-medicate, you should know what you are taking, why you are taking it, how it works, and how to use the medicines wisely.

A huge number of nonprescription medicine products are offered for sale to the public, representing about 500 active ingredients. An estimated $8 billion is spent on such products each year in the United States. There, nearly 75% of the public receives its education on OTC medicines solely from TV, radio, newspaper, and magazine advertising. Unfortunately, many of the claims for medicines are either not true or subtly misleading.

You need to be aware of the barrage of medicine advertising aimed at you. The implicit message of such advertising is that for every symptom, every ache and pain, every problem, there is a product solution. While many of the OTC products are effective, many are simply a waste of your money and a diversion of your attention from better ways of managing your illness.

If you self-medicate, here are some suggestions:

- *Always read medicine labels and patient information leaflets and follow directions carefully.* The label must by law include names and quantities of the active ingredients, precautions, and adequate directions for safe use. Careful reading of the information, including review of the individual ingredients, may help prevent you from ingesting medicines that have caused problems for you in the past. If you don't understand the dosage information on the label, ask a pharmacist before buying it.

- *Do not exceed the recommended dosage or length of treatment* unless discussed with your doctor/pharmacist.

- *Use caution if you are taking other medicines.* Over-the-counter and prescription medicines can interact, either canceling or exaggerating the effects of other medicines or alcohol. If you have questions about medicine interactions, ask your doctor or pharmacist before taking them together.

- If possible try to *select medicines with single active ingredients* rather than combination ("all-in-one") products. In using a product with multiple ingredients, you are likely to be getting medicines for symptoms you don't even have, so why risk the side effects of medicines you don't need? Single-ingredient products also allow you to adjust the dosage of each medicine separately for optimal symptom relief with minimal side effects.

- When choosing medicines, *learn the ingredient names* and try to *buy generic products*. Generics contain the same active ingredient as the brand name product, usually at a lower cost.

- *Never take or give a medicine from an unlabeled container* or a container whose label you cannot read. Keep your medicines in their original labelled containers or transfer them to a labelled medicine organiser or pill dispenser. Do not make the mistake of mixing different medicines in the same bottle.

- *Do not take medicines left over* from a previous illness or that were prescribed for someone else, even if you have similar symptoms. Always check out medicines with your doctor/pharmacist.

183

- Pills can sometimes get stuck in the oesophagus, the "feeding tube". To help prevent this, be sure to *drink at least a half glass of water* with your pills and remain standing or sitting upright for a few minutes after swallowing. (Some fruit juices interact with some medicines, so water is best.)

- If you are pregnant or nursing, have a chronic disease, or are already taking multiple medicines, *consult your pharmacist or doctor* before self-medicating.

184

- *Store your medicines in a safe place* away from the reach of any children. Poisoning with medicines is a common and preventable problem. The bathroom is not a particularly good place to store medicines. The atmosphere is often steamy and medicines should be kept dry. Consider a small, lockable tool chest or fishing box.

- Many medicines have an expiry date of about two to three years. *Discard all expired medicines by taking them to the pharmacy for safe disposal.* They should not be flushed away as some chemicals are best kept out of the water systems.

Medicines can help or harm. What often makes the difference is the care you exercise and the partnership you develop with your doctor and your pharmacist.

• • •

Suggested Further Reading

Blair, Pat. *Know Your Medicines*. London: Age Concern Books, 1997.

Henry, John A. *BMA Medicines and Drugs*, 5th ed. London: Dorling Kindersley, 2000.

Henry, John A. *The British Medical Association's Concise Guide to Medicines and Drugs*. London: Dorling Kindersley, 2001.

CHAPTER 12

Planning for the Future: Fears and Reality

P EOPLE WITH CHRONIC ILLNESSES OFTEN WORRY about what will happen to them if their disease becomes really disabling. They fear that at some time in the future they may have problems managing their lives and their illness. One way people can deal with fears of the future is to take control and plan for it. They may never need to put their plans into effect, but there is reassurance in knowing that they will still be in control if the events they fear come to pass. Here are the most common concerns and some suggestions that may be useful.

What If I Can't Take Care of Myself Anymore?

Becoming helpless and dependent is one of the most common fears among people with a potentially disabling health problem. This fear usually has physical as well as financial, social, and emotional components.

Physical Concerns of Day-to-Day Living

As your health condition changes over time, you may need to consider changing your living situation. These changes may involve hiring someone to help you in your home, negotiating with your social services department, or moving to a living situation where help is provided. The decision about which possibility is best, will be related to your needs and how best these can be met.

The first thing you will need to do is carefully *evaluate what you can do for yourself* and what activities of daily living (ADLs) will require some kind of help. ADLs are the everyday things like getting out of bed, bathing, dressing, preparing and eating your meals, cleaning house, shopping, paying bills, and so on. Most people can do all of these, even though they may have to do them slowly, with some modification or with some help from gadgets.

Some people, though, may eventually find one or more of these no longer possible without help from somebody else. For example, you may still be able to fix meals, but your mobility may be impaired to the degree that shopping is no longer possible. Or, if you have problems with fainting or sudden bouts of unconsciousness, you might need to have somebody around at all times. Using the problem-solving steps discussed in Chapter 1, analyse and make a list of what the potential problems might be. Once you have this list, problem-solve the problems one at a time, first making a list of every possible solution you can think of.

Example:

Can't go shopping

- Get son/daughter to shop for me
- Find a volunteer shopping service
- Shop at a store that delivers
- Ask neighbour to shop for me when she does her own shopping
- Get meals-on-wheels

Can't be by myself

- Hire a full-time attendant
- Move in with a relative
- Get a local council emergency response system
- Move to a residential care home
- Move to a retirement community

When you have listed your problems, and the possible solutions to the problems, select the solution that seems the most workable, acceptable, and least expensive for your needs (step 3 of problem solving).

The selection will depend upon your finances, the family or other resources you can call on, and how well any of the potential solutions will in fact solve your problem. Sometimes, one solution will be the answer for several problems. For instance, if you can't shop, can't be alone, and maybe household chores are reaching the point of a foreseeable need for help, you might consider that a retirement home will solve all of these problems, since it offers meals, regular house cleaning, and transportation for errands and medical appointments.

Even if you are not of "retirement" age, many facilities accept younger people, depending on the facility's particular policies. Most facilities for the "retired" take residents as young as 50, or younger if one of a couple is the minimum age. If you are a young person, social services disability section or "independent living centre" should be able to direct you to a local day-care facility appropriate for you.

Your appraisal of your situation and needs may be aided by sitting down with a trusted friend or relative and discussing your abilities and limitations with him or her. Sometimes another person can spot things we ourselves overlook or would like to ignore. A good self-manager often utilises other resources, which is step 6 in the problem-solving steps in Chapter 1.

Make changes in your life slowly, incrementally. You don't need to change your whole life around to solve one problem. Remember, too, that you can always change your mind if you don't burn your bridges behind you. If you think that moving out of your own place to another living arrangement (relatives, care home, etc.) would be the thing to do, don't give up your present home until you are settled in to your new home and are sure you want to stay there.

If you think you need help with some activities, hiring a home-help is less drastic than moving out and may be enough for quite a while. If you can't be alone, and you live with a family member who is away from home during the day, maybe going to an Age Concern or social services approved day centre will be enough to keep you safe and comfortable while your family is away. In fact, adult day care centres are ideal places to find new friends and activities geared to your abilities.

A social worker at your local social services department or hospital social services department can be very helpful in providing information about resources in your community and also in giving you ideas about how to deal with your care needs. There are several kinds of professionals who can be of great help. As previously mentioned, *social workers* and *health visitors* are good for helping you decide how to solve financial and living arrangement problems and locating appropriate community resources. Some social workers are also trained in counselling disabled people and/or older people in relation to emotional and relationship problems that may be associated with your health problem.

An *occupational therapist* can assess your daily living needs and suggest assistive devices or rearrangements in your home environment to make life easier.

A Disabled Employment Advisor at the Local Job Centre can help with your working environment if you are employed.

A *solicitor specialising in the law for older people* should be on your list for helping you set your financial affairs in order to preserve your assets, to prepare a proper will, and perhaps to execute an enduring or temporary power of attorney for both health care and financial management. If finances are a concern, ask your local Citizens' Advice Bureau (CAB) for the names of solicitors who offer free or low-cost services to older people. Your local Law Society can also refer you to a list of solicitors who are competent in this area. These solicitors are generally familiar with the laws applying to younger persons with disabilities as well. Even if you are not a "senior citizen", your legal needs are much the same as those of the older person.

Finding Help at Home

If you find that you cannot manage alone, the first option that comes to most people's minds is to hire some help. In fact it is a better idea to find out what is being offered by your social services department. Many of their services are not free, but they have quality standards you can keep an eye on. There are schemes for people on low incomes. Social services have a duty to support disabled people and have sections devoted to this (quite often paired up with services to older people).

You have a right to ask for an assessment of your needs. This does not mean you have to accept the services they eventually offer, but it does give you a valuable starting point. The services offered are usually focussed on making it possible for you to stay in your own home. The services available for disabled people routinely include adaptations to houses (private or council owned); equipment loan; meals on wheels; transport schemes; homecare services, advice and counselling, disabled parking badges, and usually, telephones for people who are housebound. Most will also be able to offer advice on state benefits. (This is not the case in Scotland.) Some also offer holiday schemes.

So, the first thing to do if you are coming to the conclusion that you need help at home, is to talk to social services. If you phone and ask for the duty officer you can either arrange an appointment at the office or arrange a home visit. Home care services include personal care that does not amount to nursing care. This might include helping you to get up and bathed in the morning and helping you to bed at night. Most of us do not want to admit we need this degree of help. The important thing is to come to a reasoned view long before you are approaching a crisis.

Gradually the links between social service and health service nursing support are getting closer and closer. Home carers (they have different titles in different authorities) are a vital source of information and a link to other services.

If you come to a decision that you need help in this way do not forget that you also need breaks, holidays and contact with your friends. These are part of life and it is perfectly reasonable to ask for help to maintain your activities.

Other resources that may provide help at home include Age Concern day centres and other local organisations. Age Concern or the CAB (Citizens' Advice Bureau) will know what's available. They often have listings of local services both professional and voluntary. In order to work with older people the staff have to be screened by the local police.

Finding Out-of-Home Care

Increasingly, as care available in the home through informal carers is decreasing, there are a number of options people have to find care services outside the home, but not at a great distance from it. Some of these facilities include:

Day Centres: Some people find that using the day centre services provided by local authorities and voluntary organisations can provide friendship and open doors to new activities or support. If you contact your local authority social services department, they will be able to tell you about the day centres in your area. Some will be run directly by the local authority and others by local groups such as charities for older people, church groups or different ethnic minority groups. The organised activities are often interesting and you may want to become involved in helping others while you are there. You will also meet other people there who may have similar problems as you and who could provide information on health and social services relevant to you. Day centres have their own transport services to take you to and from home.

Retirement Communities: Retirement Communities are becoming more popular and may be worth thinking about if you need little personal care but want to live in a protected area with security and emergency response services and are over 50. The communities are made up of owned or rented properties with an additional service charge. Some provide extra services, such as social facilities or nursing care for a fee. There are waiting lists for retirement communities. Some are ready to be occupied even before the building is complete. If you want to go for this option, you should register as soon as you have made the decision.

Sheltered Housing: Special Housing Associations provide sheltered housing. You will live in your own small house or flat and remain in control of how you run your life but you will be seen every day by the manager or warden and will have access to emergency support. Social events and meals are often arranged. Almshouses are available for some people on a low income or who have links with certain craft guilds. Some of these can be beautiful old cottages. Sheltered housing is not like residential care and the responsibility for your daily life will be your own.

Residential Care Homes

Residential care homes provide non-medical care and supervision for people who can't live alone. All homes (including Private Voluntary Homes) have to comply with the national minimum standards of the National Care Standards Commission (see www.doh.gov.uk/nssc/).

Residential care is not cheap and to get help with the costs you will have to have a social services assessment. Some homes are very small and some are large institutions. The services include: all meals; help with bathing and dressing; laundry; housekeeping; making arrangements for medical appointments and help with taking medicines.

You can use residential homes for short breaks to allow you to recover your strength or to give carers a break. This can also allow you to try out different local homes before you make a decision about making a lasting move because you need to find a home where you fit in. Find out about the other residents of the home to see if they are likely to be good companions. Make sure the meals are to your liking and suit your ethnic background and any dietary needs. A good home will give you as much freedom as you want and support your independence.

Nursing Homes

Nursing homes provide care for very ill or disabled people who need skilled nursing care. Nearly all come under the National Care Standards Commission as Private Voluntary Homes. Someone who has had a stroke for example, will be transferred from a hospital to a nursing home before going home. Many people are likely to spend a short time in a nursing home under Intermediate Care schemes.

The services nursing homes provide are given by qualified nurses who can manage the care of wounds, feeding tubes, respirators or other high-tech care equipment. Care from other health professionals such as physiotherapists, occupational therapists and speech therapists is also provided. A permanent nursing home patient would usually require help to get in and out of bed, eating, bathing, or managing continence.

Some nursing home specialise in certain types of care or therapy. The hospital social work department can give you advice about selecting a nursing home if you are being discharged from hospital.

Meeting the Costs of Care

Many people are afraid they will not have enough money to pay for their needs. Mostly these will be cost of equipment, services delivered to your own home, or the possible cost of residential home care. You need to start by getting a full assessment of your state benefits entitlement. Lawyers who are experts in this area often give their time as volunteers to Law Centres where you can go for professional advice. You can also get expert advice from Independent Welfare Rights Advice agencies; Citizens' Advice Bureaus with a welfare rights section; and in local authority welfare rights departments.

If you are looking for advice from your local authority welfare rights unit (please note that this service does not exist in Scotland) you need to make sure that you can find someone who can do an assessment of your benefit entitlement. Some welfare rights advisors do not do this kind of work, their job is to make sure that users of services pay something towards the cost of social services.

If you have a relative who will be your executor, you could develop a joint expertise in this area by getting the necessary information together. If you want to explore this field for yourself, the key publication is the Disability Rights Handbook. This is published each year by the Disability Alliance. For details phone 020 7247 8776. Make sure you have the latest edition if you use a library copy.

I Need Help, But Don't Want Help. Now What?

Let's talk about the emotional aspects of becoming dependent. Every human being emerges from childhood reaching for and cherishing every possible sign of independence—the driver's licence, the first job, the first bank account, the first time we go out and don't have to tell anybody where we are going or when we will be back, and so on. In these, and many other ways, we demonstrate to ourselves as well as to others that we are "grown up"—in charge of our lives and able to take care of ourselves without any help from parents.

If a time comes when we must face the realisation that we need help, that we can no longer manage completely on our own, it may seem like a return to childhood and having to let somebody else be in charge of our lives. This can be very painful and embarrassing.

Some people in this situation become extremely depressed and can no longer find any joy in life. Others fight off the recognition of their need for help, thus placing themselves in possible danger and making life difficult and frustrating for those who would like to be helpful. Still others give up completely and expect others to take total responsibility for their lives, demanding attention and services from their children or other family members. If you are having one or more of these reactions, you can help yourself to feel better and develop a more positive response.

The concept, *". . .change the things I can change, and accept the things I cannot change, and have the wisdom to know the difference,"* is really fundamental to being able to stay in charge of our lives. You must be able to correctly evaluate your situation. You must identify those activities requiring the help of somebody else (going shopping, cleaning house, for instance) and those activities you can still do on your own (getting dressed, paying bills, writing letters).

This means making decisions, and as long as you keep the decision-making prerogative, you are in charge. It is important to make decisions and take action while you are able to do so, before circumstances intervene and decisions get made for you. That means being realistic and honest with yourself.

Some people find that talking with a sympathetic listener, either a professional counsellor or a sensible close friend or family member, is very comforting and helpful. An objective listener often helps by pointing out alternatives and options you may have overlooked or were not aware of. She or he can provide information, or another point of view or interpretation of a situation that you would not have come upon yourself. This is part of the self-management process.

Be very careful, however, in evaluating advice from somebody who has something to sell you. There are many people whose solution to your problem just happens to be whatever it is they happen to be selling—funeral insurance policies, special and expensive furniture, "sunshine cruises," special magazines, or health foods with magical curative properties.

In talking with family members or friends who offer to be helpful, be as open and reasonable as you can be and, at the same time, try to make them understand that you will reserve for yourself the right to decide how much and what kind of help you will accept. They will probably be more cooperative and understanding if you can say, "Yes, I do need some help with . . . , but I still want to do . . . myself." More tips on asking for help can be found in Chapter 7, "Communicating."

Insist on being consulted. Lay the ground rules with your helpers early on. Ask to be presented with choices so that you can decide what is best for you as you see it. If you try to objectively weigh the suggestions made to you, and don't dismiss every option out of hand, people will consider you able to make reasonable decisions and will continue to provide you with the opportunity to do so.

Be appreciative. Recognize the good will and the efforts of those who want to help. Even though you may be embarrassed, you will maintain your dignity by accepting with grace the help that is offered, if you need it. If you are truly convinced that you are being offered help you don't need, you can decline it with tact and appreciation. For example, you can say, "I appreciate your offer to have Christmas at your house, but I'd like to continue having it here. I could really use some help, though—maybe with the washing-up after dinner."

If you are at length unable to come to terms with your increasing need to be dependent on others for help in managing your living situation, you might consult a professional counsellor. This should be someone who has experience with the emotional and social issues of people with disabling health problems.

Your local agency providing services to the disabled should be able to refer you to the right kind of counsellor. The local or national organization dedicated to serving people with your specific health condition (British Lung Foundation, British Heart Foundation, Diabetes UK, etc.) can also refer you to support groups and classes to help you in dealing with your condition. You should be able to locate the agency you need through the Yellow Pages under the listing "social service organisations."

Akin to the fear and embarrassment of becoming physically dependent is the fear of being abandoned by family members who would be expected to provide needed help. Tales of being "dumped" in a nursing home by children who never come to visit haunt many who worry that may happen to them.

We need to be sure that we do reach out to family and friends and ask for the help we need when we recognise that we can't go on alone. It sometimes happens that in the expectation of rejection people fail to ask for help. Some people try to hide their need in fear that their need will cause loved ones to withdraw. Families often complain, "If we'd only known . . . ," when it is revealed that a loved one had needs for help that were unmet or not known about soon enough.

If you really cannot turn to close family or friends because they are unable or unwilling to become involved in your care, there are agencies dedicated to providing for such situations. Through your local social services department you should be able to locate a "case manager" who will be able to organize the resources in your community to provide the help you need. The hospital social services department can also put you in touch with the right agencies.

Grieving—A Normal Reaction to Bad News

When we experience any kind of a loss—small ones (such as losing one's car keys) or big ones (such as losing a life partner or facing a disabling or terminal illness)—we go through an emotional process of grieving and coming to terms with the loss.

A person with a chronic, disabling health problem experiences a variety of losses. These include loss of confidence, loss of self-esteem, loss of independence, loss of the lifestyle we knew and cherished, and, perhaps the most painful of all, the loss of a positive self-image if our condition has an effect on appearance (such as rheumatoid arthritis or the residual paralysis from a stroke).

Elizabeth Kübler-Ross, who has written extensively about this process, describes the stages of grief:

193

- *Shock,* when one feels both a mental and a physical reaction to the initial recognition of the loss
- *Denial,* when the person tells himself, "No, it can't be true", and proceeds to act for a time as if it were not true
- *Anger,* the "why me?" feelings and searching for someone or something to blame (if the doctor had diagnosed it early enough I'd have been cured, or the job caused me too much stress, etc.)
- *Bargaining,* when we say to ourselves, to someone else, to God, "I'll never smoke again", or "I'll follow my treatment regimen absolutely to the letter", or "I'll go to church every Sunday, if only I can get over this"
- *Depression,* when the real awareness sets in, we confront the truth about the situation and experience deep feelings of sadness and hopelessness
- *Acceptance,* when we eventually recognize that we must deal with what has happened and make up our minds to do what we have to do

We do not pass through these stages in a linear out-of-one-into-the-next fashion. We are more apt to have several, or even many flip-flops back and forth between them. Don't be discouraged if you find yourself angry or depressed again, when you thought you had reached acceptance.

Let's talk more about the depression stage of the grief process, since this is the stage where many people get stuck, and there are several ways to move out of this stage toward acceptance.

I'm Afraid of Dying

Fear of dying is something most of us begin to experience only when something happens to bring us face to face with the possibility of our own death. Losing someone close, an accident that might have been fatal, or learning we have a health condition that may shorten our lives usually causes us to consider the inevitability of our own eventual passing. Many people, even then, try to avoid facing the future because they are afraid to think about it.

Our attitudes about death are shaped by our own central attitudes about life. This is the product of our culture, our family's influences, perhaps by our religion, and certainly by our life experiences.

If you are ready to think about your own future—about the near or distant prospect that your life will most certainly end at some time—then the ideas that follow will be useful to you. If you are not ready to think about it just yet, put this aside and come back to it later.

As with depression, the most useful way to come to terms with your eventual death is to take positive steps to prepare for it. This means to get your house in order by attending to all the necessary small and large details. If you continue to avoid dealing with these details, you will create problems for yourself and for those involved with your situation in a significant way.

The are several components to getting your house in order:

- *Decide, and then convey to others* your wishes about how and where you want to be during your last days and hours. Do you want to be in a hospital or at home? When do you want procedures to prolong your life stopped? At what point do you want to let nature take its course when it is determined that death is inevitable? Who should be with you; only the few people who are nearest and dearest, or all the people you care about and want to see one last time?

- *Make a will.* Even if your estate is a small one, you may have definite preferences about who should have what. If you have a large estate, the tax implications of a proper will may be very significant.

- *Make arrangements,* or at least plans, for your funeral. Your grieving family would be very relieved not to have to decide what you would want and how much to spend. There are prepaid "future need" funeral plans available, and you can purchase burial space where and of the type you prefer.

- *Make an enduring power of attorney for health care,* and also one that will let someone manage your financial affairs. You should also discuss your wishes with your GP, even if he or she doesn't seem to be very interested. (Your GP may also have trouble facing the prospect of losing you.) This is discussed in Chapter 9.

195

Be sure that some kind of document or notation is included in your medical records that indicates your wishes in case you can't communicate them when the time comes.

Be sure that the persons you want to handle things after your death (your executor[s])are *aware of all that they need to know* about your wishes, your plans and arrangements, and the location of necessary documents. You will need to talk to them, or at least prepare a detailed letter of instructions, and give it to someone who can be counted on to deliver it to the proper person when needed. This should be a person close enough to you to know when that time is at hand. You may not want your spouse to have to take on these responsibilities, for example, but your spouse may be the best person to keep your letter and know when to give it to your designated agent.

At any well-stocked stationery store you can purchase a pre-organised kit, in which you place a copy of your will, important papers, and information about your financial and personal affairs. There are forms that you fill out about bank and charge accounts, insurance policies, the location of important documents, your safe deposit box and where the key is kept, and so on. This is a handy, concise way of getting everything together that anyone might need to know about.

- *Finish "business" with the world around you.* Mend your relationships. Pay your debts, both financial and personal. Say what needs to be said to those who need to hear it. Do what needs to be done. Forgive yourself. Forgive others.

- *Talk about your feelings about your death.* Most family and close friends are reluctant to initiate such a conversation, but appreciate it if you bring it up. You may find that there is much to say and to hear from your loved ones. If you find that they are unwilling to listen to you talk about your death and the feelings that you are perceiving, find someone who will be comfortable and empathetic in listening to you. Your family and friends may be able to listen to you later on. Remember, those who love you will also go through the stages of grieving when they have to think about the prospect of losing you.

A large component in fear of death is the fear of the unknown. "What will it be like?" "Will it be painful?" "What will happen to me (after I die)?"

Most people who die of a disease are ready to die when the time comes. Painkillers and the disease process itself weaken body and mind, and the awareness of self diminishes without the realization that this is happening. Most people just "slip away," with the transition between the state of living and that of no longer living hardly identifiable. Reports from people who have been brought back to life after being in a state of clinical death indicate they experienced a sense of peacefulness and clarity and were not frightened.

However, a dying person may sometimes feel very lonely and abandoned. Regrettably, many people cannot deal with their own emotions when they are around a person they know to be dying and so deliberately avoid his or her company, or they may engage in superficial chitchat, broken by long awkward silences.

This is often puzzling and hurtful to those who are dying, who need companionship and solace from those they counted on.

You can sometimes help by telling your family and friends what you want and need from them—attention, entertainment, comfort, practical help, and so on. Again, when a person has something positive to do, they are more able to cope with their emotions. If you can engage your family and loved ones in specific activities, they can feel needed and can relate to you around the activity. This will give you something to talk about, to occupy time, or it will at least provide a definition of the situation for them and for you.

If you choose to die at home, the support of a local hospice can be very helpful. These organisations provide both physical and emotional care to people who are dying, as well as for their families. The local hospice may be able to arrange for setting up your home to meet your needs and take care of the details of your care both before and at the time of death. This can be a great help to loved ones. To find a hospice near you, ask the hospital social worker or your doctor.

Hospice care, as with everything else discussed in this chapter, can be arranged before the time it's needed. Planning ahead can be a comfort to both you and your loved ones.

• • •

Suggested Further Reading

American Heart Association. *American Heart Association Guide to Heart Attack, Treatment, Recovery, and Prevention.* New York: Times Books, 1998.

Callahan, Maggie, and Patricia Kelley. *Final Gifts: Understanding the Special Awareness, Needs, and Communications of the Dying.* New York: Bantam Books, 1997.

Copeland, Mary Ellen, and Wayne London. *The Depression Workbook: A Guide for Living with Depression and Manic Depression.* Oakland, Calif.: New Harbinger Publications, 1992.

Gilbert, Paul. *Overcoming Depression.* Constable Robinson, 2000.

Kübler-Ross, Elizabeth. *On Death and Dying.* New York: Scribner Classics, 1997.

Lewinsohn, Peter M., editor. *Control Your Depression.* Simon & Schuster, 1992.

Whybrow, Ruth. *Caring for Elderly Parents.* Crossroads Publishers, 1996.

Wilkinson, James A. *A Family Caregiver's Guide to Planning and Decision Making for the Elderly.* Minneapolis, Minn.: Fairview Publishing, 1999.

CHAPTER
13

Helpful Hints

T HERE ARE MANY WAYS TO ORGANISE YOUR LIFE AND PEOPLE OFTEN CREATE "SHORTCUTS" TO MAKE THINGS EASIER. Here are a few tips. These suggestions are offered to stimulate your imagination and problem-solving abilities. Not everything works for everyone. Use what is helpful.

You may find it helpful to visit a Disabled Living Centre where you can get advice on equipment. There are many centres across the UK and their website has addresses and phone numbers: www.dlcc.org.uk

Waking Up

- Try some stretching and strengthening exercises while you are still in bed.

- A duvet can replace a bedspread and is easy to pull up.

- Do some of your dressing sitting on the edge of your bed before you get up. Leave the clothes within reach of your bed the night before.

- While you are still in bed, warm your bed with a hot water bottle just before you do your exercise to help loosen morning stiffness.

- Keep a walking stick or chair next to your bed to help pull yourself out of bed in the morning.

Bathing

- If you find standing in a shower or sitting down in the bath difficult, get a bath stool. It is waterproof and fits in the bath. You can sit while you bathe.

- Replace shower heads or bath taps with a hand-held sprayer unit.

- If you are feeling weak, a "sponge bath" can be taken in place of a full bath and can be a lot less taxing.

- Using a long, absorbent, cotton terry robe cuts out the effort of drying with a towel.

- Soap on a rope lets you use soap with one hand, and keeps it from falling.

- A liquid soap dispenser may be easier to use than a bar of soap.

- Replace difficult twist tops on shampoo or lotions with pump tops.

- A shower caddy keeps bathing supplies within easy reach.

- Use non-skid safety strips or a rubber bath mat in the bath or shower.

- Consider having grab bars installed in your bath or shower to reduce the risk of falling.

- Get a long-handled sponge or brush.

- Suctioned soap holders make it possible to soap yourself without grasping the soap or needing to use two hands.

Looking after Your Teeth

- Suctioned brushes are useful for cleaning dentures with one hand.

- Electric toothbrushes make brushing easier.

- Get a dental-floss holder if flossing is difficult with two hands.

- Look for toothpaste in pumps rather than tubes. The heel of one hand can press the pump.

- Look for special long or curved handled toothbrushes.

- Toothbrush handles can be made easier to grasp by wrapping a small sponge or foam hair curler around them.

Female Hygiene

- Hand-held female urinals make it possible for a woman to urinate standing up.

- Women who sometimes accidentally pass urine find that small panty liners or sanitary pads with adhesive backs help avoid embarrassment.

- Women who use pads for periods can keep the genital area clean using a squeeze bottle of water kept by the toilet. These bottles can be found with a variety of spray nozzles.

Grooming

- A small sponge around the handle of a razor or an eyeliner pencil can make them easier to grasp.

- Long handled brushes and combs make it easier to reach hair.

- Shaving or applying make-up is easier if you have a mirror set low enough for you to sit down.

- If you have respiratory problems, switch to non-aerosol toiletries. You can get liquid hair dressings and roll-on deodorants. You can also get unscented toiletries.

Dressing

- Lower the rod in your wardrobe or get a wardrobe organiser to bring clothes within easier reach.

- If balance or mobility are problems, it is safer and easier to pull underpants and trousers up when lying in bed.

- When you shop for clothes, look for easy-to-reach fasteners, front openings, and elastic waistbands loose enough to be pulled over the hips.

- Look for clothes with Velcro or elastic instead of buttons.

- Replace the buttons on your garments with Velcro. Move the buttons to the top part of the opening for decoration.

- Bras can be fastened in front and then turned around and pulled into place, or buy front-opening bras.

- Dusting powder on the thighs makes pulling on tights easier.

- Most women find that wearing trousers and socks is much easier than struggling into tights.

- Put rings or loops on zip fasteners to make it easier to pull zips.

- If hot or cold temperatures bother you, you may find cotton underclothing more comfortable than synthetic.

- Use a bent coat hanger to help with retrieving clothes that are out of reach.

- Get a long-handled shoehorn.

- Slip-on shoes are easy and require no bending over to tie, convert lace-up shoes to slip-ons with elastic shoelaces.

- When shopping for clothes, take a tape measure with you that is marked with your measurements. By measuring the garments, you may not have to try on so many before you buy.

- Choose women's trousers or skirts with pockets, and carry money, driver's license, and so on, in the pockets instead of carrying a large, heavy handbag.

Getting Around

- Lead with your strongest leg when going up stairs. Lead with your weaker leg when going down.

- Remove all throw rugs—they can cause falls.

- Doorways inside your home can be made wider by removing the doors, making them easier to get through with a wheelchair, walking aid, or other equipment.

- Consider installing stair rails on both sides of the stairway to increase safety.

- A small ramp can replace a couple of stairs at the entrance to your home or elsewhere. (Be careful of building regulations, though!)

- Carry a folding walking chair seat with you when you go out. It gives you both something to lean on and something to sit on when necessary.

- Place a chair or table near the top of stairs to lean or sit on when you reach the top.

- To lift and carry:
  1. Lift or carry while exhaling through pursed lips.
  2. Rest and inhale through nose; continue this pattern of intermittent work and rest until you get the job done.

Doing Household Chores

- Get a small serving trolley; some fold, most have two shelves. As you do the household chores, use the trolley to carry your supplies or things that need to be put away. If you live in a two-storey house, keep a trolley on each level.

- Reachers can retrieve things from hard-to-reach places. Reachers can be bought from Boots and most other medical supply shops.

- A magnet tied to a string can help pick up drawing pins, hairpins, and so on. It will stick to your trolley, refrigerator or washing machine.

- Long-handled sponges are good for hard to reach areas such as your bath.

- Consider a battery-powered "scrubber" for bathtub, sink, and so on.

- Get a long-handled dustpan and a small broom for dry spills.

- Foam floor mats can be placed where you may need to stand often, such as at the sink, ironing board, or telephone. They can reduce foot and ankle pain and low back pain.

- Use an adjustable-height ironing board so that you can sit down while ironing.

- Small items such as socks or underwear can be washed in laundry bags to avoid having to search in the washer or dryer.

- Use gravity to get clothes out of the dryer or front-loading washer. Put a basket under the door and scoop the clothes into it with a reacher or stick.

- Try old-fashioned push-on clothespegs rather than pinch clothespegs.

- Fitted bed sheets are difficult to put on the bed, slit one corner and fasten with a tie.

- Use a large, wide spatula to tuck in sheets.

- Use a vacuum cleaner with disposable bags, but remember if you have respiratory problems to remove the bag with extreme care.

- A small, battery-powered hand vacuum is easy to use for spot clean-ups and can be kept on your trolley.

- A damp cloth is good for dusting. If you don't want to use anything damp on wood surfaces, get a roll of paper towels and a bottle of lemon oil. Put 4 or 5 dots of oil on each towel, use and throw away.

- People with respiratory problems should not use aerosol cleaning products.

- Avoid substances that can vaporise, such as mothballs, solvents, and kerosene.

Cooking, Eating and Kitchen Stuff

- Microwaves save time and energy.

- Replace the twist-ties on bread or other foods with clothespegs.

- Avoid lifting heavy pots of food along with the water they were cooked in. Place food in a basket to lower into the water for cooking, or get a spaghetti cooker with holes in. Lift the basket out to drain food. Someone else can drain the pot later, or you can ladle it out.

- Ask family members not to close jars too tightly. A jar opener can be mounted under a countertop, or you can get a rubber disk to help you open jars.

- Don't try to get everything done at once. Almost all jobs can be divided into small tasks. For instance, clean the top shelf of the refrigerator today and the bottom shelf tomorrow.

- Place on one of your kitchen shelves a water container that has a tap near the bottom so that you won't have to lift the container to fill your drinking glass.

- Cook double or triple quantities of the recipe. Freeze the extra portions in meal-sized containers. In a microwave, they can be easily thawed and heated without drying out.

- A slow-cooker can make many meals easier to prepare, as can a pressure cooker.

- Always use an extractor fan when cooking, especially if you have respiratory problems.

- A small, portable fan can help you overcome shortness of breath or cool you off in a warm kitchen. Some are battery-powered and can clip on to a shelf.

- Use a trolley when tidying up after a meal. Gather all the items that need to go into the refrigerator, and then sit down with the trolley and put them away all at once.

- Put your most used pots and pans back on the cooker and leave them there. Instead of putting dishes and cutlery away, reset the table for the next meal.

- Try a serving dish with spikes sticking up that will hold meat firmly in place while you cut it. If necessary, you will be able to carve meat with one hand.

- Put flour and sugar in conveniently located containers so that you won't have to lift the heavy bags.

- Oven gloves allow you to lift hot pans with both hands.

- A pizza wheel can cut it easily!

- A small food processor can make grating, chopping, or slicing easier.

- Wheeled stools in the kitchen will make work easier . . . at counter height or low enough to allow you to get into lower cabinets with minimal bending.

- While eating If you have difficulty using a knife, try a pizza cutter to cut the food into bite-size pieces.

- Use a scoop dish with a non-skid bottom to avoid pushing food off the plate.

Remembering to Take Medicines

- A pillbox with a separate compartment for each day of the week is useful. A pillbox can be made out of an egg carton or bought at your local chemist.

- Some electronic pillboxes can be programmed to "beep" you when it's time to take your medicine.

- Combine medicine taking with a normal, daily habit, such as brushing your teeth. Put your pills next to the things you use for that activity, such as a toothbrush (making sure your medicines are out of the reach of children).

- Whenever you get a prescription, work out how long it will last and mark the time to re-order on a calendar. This may save you from running out at a weekend or holiday.

Shopping

- If you have a home computer with a modem, you can do some shopping by computer on the Internet.

- At the supermarket check out always ask for help with packing and get your fresh food items packed in a separate bag.

- Some shopping centres now offer shopability schemes with powered wheelchairs equipped with shopping trolleys.

- Mail-order catalogues offer some of the things you would want, and are fun to look through.

Going Out

- Become assertive about exposure to other people's tobacco smoke. You have a right to breathe smoke-free air. Ask smokers near you to stop.

- Wash your hands well when you get home. Colds and other diseases are often spread by touch.

- Before going out, prepare for your return home. Lay out your comfortable clothes and slippers, leave a drink in a handy thermos, set out what you will need for your evening meal.

- If you don't already have one, ask your social services department about getting a disabled parking permit. Even if you don't drive, a friend can use this when you go out together.

- If you fill the petrol tank, try to position yourself upwind so that you don't breathe in the fumes.

- When shopping for a new car, look for easily-opened doors and easily-adjusted seats. Attach a loop to the inside door handle of your car to make it easier to pull-close it.

- Get plastic extenders that make seat belts easier to get hold of if they retract to a place behind your shoulder.

- Wide-angle rear-view mirrors allow better visibility without neck strain.

- A back support device can make a car seat more comfortable.

Gardening

- A sit-in, motorised lawnmower with a self-starting mechanism, can be a real morale booster.

- Find lightweight, easy-to-handle tools.

- Use a folding stool or one with wheels. There are wheeled stools especially for gardening, with a tool storage area under the seat.

- Many tools can be purchased with a long handle, or you can have a short handle replaced with a long one.

- Build up planting beds so that you can sit on the edge and do the gardening.

208

Build Friendships

- Somewhere near you there is someone who needs your friendship and help. Look for these opportunities.

- Set up a telephone network with friends, these contacts will be able to help in case of emergency.

- Think of a signal, such as a pulled-down blind at night, to let your neighbours know you are all right.

- Home computers and digital television services are becoming more affordable. You can play long-distance board games by email.

- You can also play some games over the phone.

- Your computer can introduce you to other people through chat rooms and by e-mail. Be cautious!

- Learn to use your computer or take art classes in an adult education class in your local community. This can be a way of meeting interesting people.

- If you like to paint, consider watercolours. They are lightweight, odourless, and dry quickly.

- The Open College and the Open University offer adult education classes through television or correspondence.

- If your previous hobbies are too demanding, try scaling them down. Start a container garden or try bonsai or orchids rather than a full-sized garden.

- An embroidery frame and stand will allow you to do needlework without having to use your hands to stabilise the piece you are working on.

- Self-threading needles are available at fabric shops and through catalogues. Ask a relative to give you threaded needles for your birthday.

Travelling

- Ask your doctor about your tolerance to altitude and cabin air pressures before you travel by air. Be aware of the altitudes of your destination.

- You can arrange in advance with airlines for a wheelchair, special boarding and seating, or special meals. Be sure to confirm the arrangements at least 48 hours before your flight.

- Travel light. Get suitcases with well spaced wheels, or get a rolling luggage rack.

- Instead of a handbag, use a waistcoat with lots of pockets.

- Find out if there is a travel agent in your area who specialises in travel for people with physical impairments.

Getting Sleep

- Go to bed in stages so that you arrive relaxed, not worn out. Put on your nightclothes and then relax by reading or watching television for a little while. Have everything you need near your bed, such as a telephone and a light. Have emergency numbers attached to the phone, or use a phone with an auto-dial feature.

- A night-light will help prevent falls or feeling disorientated in the dark.

- Keep a torch near the bed for emergencies.

- Bedtime is often a good time to do some gentle muscle-relaxation exercises.

Keeping Warm

- Heating pads come in a many shapes and sizes, to fit just about any part of your body.

- Soak stiff, sore hands or feet in warm water.

- Thermoelastic gloves are good for warming. They are available at some chemists. Thermoeleastic products are also available for knees and elbows.

- Electric blankets and electric mattress pads are lightweight and warm.

- Sleeping inside a sleeping bag placed under a blanket will help to keep you warm.

- Consider wearing long underwear. It comes in many colours and styles.

- A large shawl is good for the occasional shivers, and much easier to put on and take off then a sweater.

210

• • •

Suggested Further Reading

Biegel, David E., Eva Kahana, and May Wykle. *Family Caregiving Across the Lifespan.* Sage Publications Inc., 1994.

Schwarz, Shelly. *300 Tips for Making Life with Multiple Sclerosis Easier.* Demos Medical Publishing, 1999.

INDEX

213

214